GW01393106

A graduate of IIT Delhi, Anil Bhatnagar worked with SAIL for twenty-one years before quitting his job to dedicate his life to all he was born for—Reiki, writing, lecturing, painting, poetry and coaching people and corporations on how to grow and thrive rather than just survive. He is now an experienced Reiki teacher, corporate trainer, motivational speaker, personal-growth coach and a pioneer in spiritualizing corporate operations. He is the author of several books, including *Ten Keys to Corporate and Personal Success*, *Water the Roots* and *The Little Book of Forgiveness*, and he writes regularly for magazines such as *Life Positive, Training and Management* and *Executive Excellence*, a magazine published by the Covey Leadership Center in the U.S. His passion for learning drives him to study continually the wisdom of the spiritual giants of every era, and his passion for teaching takes him to corporations, colleges, schools, institutes and clubs to share his thoughts on Reiki, spiritual and emotional intelligence, spiritual growth, time management, neuro-linguistic programming, interpersonal communication, personal management, yoga, pranayama, meditation, attitudinal change and corporate success.

He feels strongly about making his humble contribution, in whatever little way he can, towards improving the conditions of orphans, old people, animals, females and Mother Earth. In 1990 he founded a free primary school in Rourkela for poor children who work as helpers in local shops.

Bhatnagar lives with his wife Aruna, a practising Reiki master, and their children Moksha and Vedant on the outskirts of Delhi. He practises Reiki, yoga, Sudarshan Kriya, tai chi and meditation regularly. Questions and suggestions can be addressed to:

Anil Bhatnagar
305, Vindhyachal Tower
Kaushambi, Ghaziabad, U.P. 201010
anil_bhatnagar_2000@yahoo.com
91/477–3384

Transform Your Life with Reiki

Anil Bhatnagar

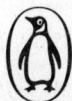

PENGUIN BOOKS

Reiki is a miraculously effective method of energy healing that brings all-around growth and development. It is transforming the lives of people all over the world. Nevertheless, Reiki and the information in this book cannot be used as a substitute for professional medical help, especially in the case of emergencies and serious diseases. Ensure that you secure the advice of your physician or another health-care professional at such times.

Kindly note as well that you cannot gain the ability to flow Reiki through your hands to heal yourself and others merely by reading this book (or any other), or by watching demonstrations or listening to lecture tapes. To learn Reiki you must approach a bona fide Reiki master and get yourself attuned. Though the information in this book is based on careful research, the author and publisher are not liable for any damage resulting directly or indirectly from its application.

PENGUIN BOOKS

Published by the Penguin Group

Penguin Books India Pvt Ltd, 11 Community Centre, Panchsheel Park, New Delhi 110 017, India

Penguin Group (USA) Inc., 375 Hudson Street, New York, New York 10014, USA

Penguin Group (Canada), 10 Alcorn Avenue, Toronto, Ontario, Canada M4V 3B2 (a division of Pearson Penguin Canada Inc.)

Penguin Books Ltd, 80 Strand, London WC2R 0RL, England

Penguin, Ireland, 25 St Stephen's Green, Dublin 2, Ireland (a division of Penguin Books Ltd)

Penguin Group (Australia), 250 Camberwell Road, Camberwell, Victoria 3124, Australia (a division of Pearson Australia Group Pty Ltd)

Penguin Group (NZ), cnr Airborne and Rosedale Road, Albany, Auckland 1310, New Zealand (a division of Pearson New Zealand Ltd)

Penguin Group (South Africa) (Pty) Ltd, 24 Sturdee Avenue, Rosebank, Johannesburg 2196, South Africa

Penguin Books Ltd, Registered Offices: 80 Strand, London WC2R 0RL, England

First published by Penguin Books India 2002

Typeset in Sabon by Mantra Virtual Services, New Delhi

Printed at Pauls Press, New Delhi

Contents

Acknowledgements

I am grateful to Reiki and my spirit guides for having awakened me to the beauty of life and given me the wonderful gift of Reiki. I am also grateful to the universe for having given me the opportunity to understand, experience, study and share this great science of Reiki and serve her thereby.

I am grateful to my parents, my brothers, my sisters and their families for being a part of my destiny and for the love they have showered on me.

I am grateful to Aruna, my wife, who gave her inputs as a true committed Reiki teacher. She encouraged me to give the five principles of Reiki the importance they deserve, and it was her idea to promote Reiki as a way of life, not merely a healing therapy. Her sincerity towards both Reiki and life has given new dimension and meaning to this book and to my life. She always wanted to see me write a book that does not ignore the sceptic, that shows the same compassion for all readers regardless of their present beliefs and convictions. If this book has come anywhere near the true spirit of Reiki, and endears itself to the reader's mind, heart and spirit, the credit goes to her.

I am grateful to Sukhdeepak Malvai, my Reiki teacher, who initiated me and my wife into all the Reiki levels, and to his masters, Shyamal Dhutve and Sandeep Joshi. I am also grateful to Dr Mikao Usui, the re-discoverer of Reiki, and to Dr Hyashi,

Madam Takata and all the other Reiki masters of the past, present and future.

I am grateful to my students and patients, from whom I have learnt a great deal, and to my daughter Moksha and my son Vedant for being true Reiki channels (second degree) and for all the love and support they gave me during the writing of this book.

I am also grateful to Penguin India, especially to Mr David Davidar and Ms V.K. Karthika for the trust they reposed in me and the book, and to Christine Cipriani for the extraordinary passion, patience, competence and sincerity with which she edited the book. Finally, I am grateful to my brother Girish Bhatnagar, who tirelessly took hundreds of digital photos to facilitate the book's illustrations.

Preface

Imagine that you are a fish. You were born in the ocean, with water all around you. Never for a moment have you been without it.

One day, all of a sudden, you are ripped out of your environment. There is not a drop of water around you. What is your immediate reaction? What do you suddenly yearn for? Water, naturally! It is your nature to be in water always. You cannot live without it.

Now come back to reality. You are a human being, not a fish. You are not yearning for water, but you are very much yearning for something else—happiness. You have sought it all your life. Why? Not because you have unreasonable expectations, but because deep down it is in your intrinsic nature to be happy. You are happiness personified! There was a time when you were surrounded by bliss and happiness on every side, like a fish is surrounded by water. One day, all of a sudden, you were ripped out of your environment. There was no sign of happiness anywhere, only darkness and struggle. Happiness became a thing of the past, and before long you forgot your true nature altogether. You still have faint memories of your true nature, but your life has become a compromise: the occasional miserly bath in fleeting pleasure, instead of the ocean of happiness that used to be your home.

But there is a difference. In the case of the fish, she really was ripped out of the water; in your case, it has only been a bad dream. You are still in the ocean of happiness. To reclaim your natural habitat you need only to wake up.

And to wake up, you have only to start believing and expecting precisely what you want to see—the ocean of happiness!

Reiki is just the right vehicle for this journey, as it facilitates our route to the forgotten oneness of which we are already a part. It will transform your personality, your relationships, your emotional life, your professional life, your creativity and enhance your sense of being unconditionally secure, cheerful and happy. Reiki ensures abundance in all aspects of your life: abundance of happiness, abundance of love for yourself and everyone else, abundance of wealth, abundance of success, abundance of creativity and abundance of gratitude.

In India we advise tourists, 'Do not make the mistake of leaving India before seeing the Taj Mahal.' And I feel like saying to everyone who happens to be a tourist on this planet, 'If you have come to Earth and been granted this beautiful life with so many possibilities, do not make the mistake of leaving without experiencing the bliss of Reiki.'

All that is pleasant and beautiful flows naturally from Reiki. Life is not the same once you introduce yourself to this new way of living—everything starts to change for the better. The time-line of your life divides clearly into pre-Reiki and post-Reiki. Desires either get fulfilled or drop away, and the mist over your purpose in life starts to clear. You begin making decisions that you have put off for years. A directionless life turns into a meaningful one, and you soon wonder how you were so fortunate as to have found the world of Reiki.

But unfortunately, the vast majority of people still opt to grapple with all kinds of problems using anything and everything but Reiki. Our concern should not be whether or not Reiki works, or how and why it works, but that so many people live on a planet blessed with the knowledge of Reiki yet go through their entire lives without hearing its name—or, if they do hear of Reiki, they disbelieve it and discard it before even trying it.

They do not deem it important enough to be given a place in their lives.

Most energy healing systems take years of study and practice to be used effectively. Imagine a system so simple that an ordinary person, who has never believed in the possibility of healing people just by the laying-on of hands, becomes a healer on the same day of his or her attunement! Reiki is a holistic energy healing system with a difference—it promises less and provides more.

My own entry into Reiki came out of sheer curiosity. I did not have very high expectations; I could not have imagined that my destiny was to become a Reiki master teacher myself. Over the last few years, I and Aruna, my wife, have watched Reiki transform not only our own lives but also those of our students and patients in profound and incredible ways. I am only a beginner—and I would love always to feel like one (Reiki is like a mother to me, and sons never grow old to a mother)—but Reiki has already transformed my life. One change is that I have learnt to be happy irrespective of external situations. I can decide to be happy at any time, under any circumstances, and nothing can stop me. My health has improved considerably. I am much more confident in myself. The very nature of my goals in life has changed. Instead of thinking, 'I will achieve this for myself,' I set goals in terms of giving to others. I have come to trust myself. A sense that I am constantly being taken care of by the higher forces of the universe permeates every cell of my body. I almost never feel insecure, financially or otherwise. Like new-found wings, freedom has started growing on me. I recently gave up my safe, secure and comfortable job of twenty-one years' standing (I still had seventeen years to go) to pursue things closer to my heart and fulfil the purpose I was born for—to learn, share and grow in Love and Truth.

Just the other day I heard someone say, 'I have heard many Reiki masters and channels talk about Reiki, but I am eager to hear the views of an outsider—someone who is not deeply "into it" but has just seen or felt it working in his own life.' I told him it is actually difficult to find such people, as those who see Reiki working cannot keep themselves 'outside' Reiki much longer. They become insiders very soon. Paula Horan, the internationally renowned Reiki master who brought Reiki to India, was once a breast-cancer patient herself.

There is a plethora of books on Reiki in the market. Some are truly informative, and discuss the subject with deep sincerity. These books have been found quite useful by those who already practise Reiki or know they want to give it a try. But what about those who do not want to try Reiki simply because they are not convinced that the energy emitted by someone's hands can heal?

There is an undercurrent of complacency in most of these books regarding the reader's preparedness to accept the very concept of Reiki. This complacency is not difficult to understand; many Reiki masters believe that we cannot prepare anyone to accept something like Reiki before their destined time or against their wish. And to a large extent, I agree. But I also believe that countless people would not object to the idea of Reiki if they could only see the logic in it. And someone has to build a bridge between their world of 'logic' and the truth from which Reiki stems, so they can cross over to the other side and feel Reiki's bliss.

Most books on Reiki also promote it as a 'healing therapy', which I believe belittles its scope. Calling Reiki a healing therapy may be a good way of letting people enter its world through the back door, but this is unjust to the spirit of Reiki. Reiki is a way of life and should be promoted as such—and that is the message and the spirit of this book.

1

The Secret Human Anatomy: The Aura

In order to understand how Reiki brings us back to our true nature, we need to understand that the body we see in the mirror and identify ourselves with is merely the tip of the iceberg.

For thousands of years we have seen pictures of great saints and holy men like Jesus Christ, Guru Nanak, Lord Buddha and Shirdi Sai Baba with haloes around their heads. Some images also show light rays emerging from their hands. As a child, I thought the depiction of a halo was just the artist's way of showing respect; haloes have become so integral to pictures of saints and godmen that we take them for granted. Haloes were considered imaginary by most people, and especially by the scientific community—until around thirty years ago, when a Russian scientist named Seymon Kirlian invented Kirlian photography, a process by which we can photograph the bioplasmic energy commonly known as the *aura*. The halo is simply the part of the aura around the head.

Kirlian photography uses a high-frequency electrical current (from a generator that produces 75,000 to 200,000 oscillations per second) instead of light to expose a film. A Kirlian picture of a living body shows a corona around it. The advent of Kirlian photography not only generated new interest but also triggered serious scientific investigation into the world of auras. Ancient Eastern scriptures that had been gathering dust were taken off the shelves and given serious study. Scientific research with the assistance of clairvoyants has revealed a correlation between the observations of these gifted people and Kirlian photography, and thus validated most of the descriptions of auras given in our scriptures.

Each human body is surrounded by one of these ever-changing, egg-shaped dynamic energy systems, and it is at this level—the invisible anatomy of the human energy field—that Reiki acts and carries out the process of healing. The energy body comes into being before the physical body, and dissipates after the physical body's death. If you cut a leaf, the bioplasmic field will continue to hold the shape and form of the complete leaf; it will take some time before assuming the truncated from. Similarly, patients whose limbs are amputated continue to feel the presence of their limbs long after the operation.

Reiki holds, and scientific research so far suggests, that all diseases first originate in the auric or energy body and get projected on to the physical plane in due time. A clean, healthy aura therefore means a healthy body. Auras can also be diagnosed with the help of pendulums or with sensitized hands. In order to sensitize your hands, rub them briskly against each other, hold them about twenty inches apart and slowly move them towards each other. Try to feel the energy building up between them. (Closing your eyes might help you focus on the sensations.) In a few days' time, you will develop a reasonable sensitivity in your hands. Ted Andrews, author of *How to See Auras with the Naked Eye*, prescribes an interesting exercise: stand behind someone at a distance just farther than that of your outstretched arms. Sway your body back and forth. Ask your partner to keep his body relaxed and loose. Ask a volunteer to observe the movements of your partner. You and the volunteer will find that your partner's body also starts moving to and fro, following your own body. These movements originate in the push and pull you are giving to your partner's energy field.

THE SEVEN KOSHAS

The auric field is composed of seven layers, each one interpenetrating and extending out from the previous one (Fig. 1).

The first layer intersperses the physical body and extends out of it by one-and-a-half to two inches. The first layer deals with the functioning of the physical body, including such physical sensations as pain, heat and cold. Our need on this level is to enjoy a healthy, vibrant body and the physical sensations associated with health. The colour of the aura on this level ranges from fine, thin, light aqua-blue for quiet and sensitive people to thick, coarse, deep bluish-grey for strong, robust people. The health of the first layer determines our potential for enjoying physical life.

The second layer represents our emotions with respect to ourselves. We need to love and accept ourselves as we are. Images for this layer range from vibrant, brightly coloured clouds (positive feelings) to dark, murky shades (negative feelings). These clouds of energy flow along the energy lines of the first layer. If you stop the flow of these feelings, you stop the flow of the clouds, and they become dark and sluggish. A stagnant second layer can impede the flow of the first and third layers.

The third layer represents logic and clarity, with which we think and desire to learn new things. The energy lines here are fine and

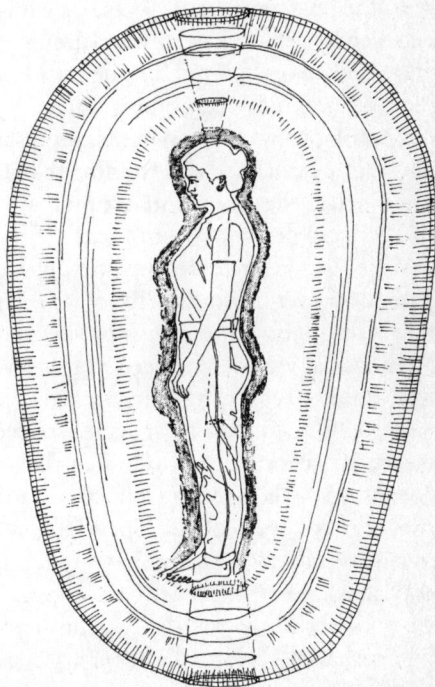

Fig. 1

thin, lemon-yellow in colour, and pulsate at a very high rate. A dull layer shows dullness of mind and disinclination to think. Negative thoughts correlate with slower pulsations of the field in this region and dark, distorted energy lines. An alert and agile mind keeps this layer healthy.

The fourth layer represents our feelings for the people we relate to. At this level, we need to love and be loved. This level is the bridge between our physical world (experienced through our first three layers) and the spiritual world (experienced through the next three). The energy here is thick and fluid, and it vibrates faster than the second layer. An unhealthy fourth layer is dark and heavy, with the consistency of mucus. The energy of the fourth layer flows between people as they interact; streams of bioplasmic energy move out from your layer towards the other person's field. These streams can be soft and rosy between lovers; dark, sticky and grey-green when one is jealous; high-peaked orange-red for one burning with passion; or dark-red and pointed when one is angry. We are born with cords connecting us with our parents, representing our relationships with our parents and determining the kinds of relationships we form with the men and women in our lives. Each new relationship develops more cords.

The fifth layer represents the divine will, and is associated with the power of words in the creative process. It is by accessing this layer that what we wish or say to ourselves comes true in the physical world. The need at this level is to be who we are, and to express that person to others. Those with an underdeveloped fifth layer have trouble keeping their lives in order; they cannot figure out their purpose in life. Those with a developed fifth layer are punctual, good planners and good executors of their plans. They have a sense of meaning and purpose in their lives, and have space and time for everything they need. The fifth level has grooves or slots for the bluish energy lines of the first layer. This kosha is the mould for the first kosha, as it creates the necessary negative space and contains all the shapes and forms that exist in the first kosha. This kosha extends one-and-a-half to two feet from the body.

The sixth layer represents divine love and ecstasy. Here are the feelings we experience when we fall in love with someone, get lost in the beauty of a landscape and so forth. Extending two to two-and-three-quarters feet from the body, the sixth kosha is a gold-silver halo of light. Our need at this level is for spiritual nourishment through experiences that make us feel lost in something — we might feel connected to the stars, the trees, the ocean or everything out there in the universe — thus giving us the experience of oneness. This is the level we experience in deep meditation. This level comprises streams of light of various colours, radiating in all directions at a high frequency. The beams may be straight or sagging, depending upon the health of this level.

The seventh layer represents the divine mind, and is made up of beautiful, high-frequency, bright golden energy lines. Extending three to three-and-a-half feet from the body, these golden lines form the matrix for all the physical components of our bodies. With a well developed seventh kosha, we start seeing and feeling the hidden divine perfection. A hidden purpose appears in every seemingly imperfect event or item around you, resulting in serenity of mind. At this level you hold your core beliefs, which may or may not be in harmony with the universal laws. All of our creative ideas flow from this level and give a sense of purpose to them. When the seventh kosha is underdeveloped, we might feel that everything is disconnected, random, chaotic and without purpose. When our beliefs are in disharmony with the divine laws, we are bound to experience diseases and upsets. This kosha holds the entire energy field together and protects it from harm.

THE SEVEN CHAKRAS

The aura is created and nourished by the energy brought in through chakras (*chakra* means 'wheel' or 'vortex' in Sanskrit), centres of nervous and cerebral energy that form the interface between the aura and the physical body. Though there are thousands of chakras throughout the human body, there are seven main energy vortices in the vicinity of their endocrine counterparts along the spine: *mooladhara* (the root chakra), *svadhisthana* (hara, or sexual chakra), *manipura* (solar-plexus chakra), *anahata* (heart chakra), *vishudha* (throat chakra), *ajna* (third-eye chakra) and, *sahasrara* (crown chakra). Their colour varies from violet at the crown chakra to red at the root chakra, just as in a rainbow. Each chakra has a different number of vortices (shown as the petals of a flower in the ancient texts), and from *mooladhara* to *sahasrara* their numbers are 4, 6, 10, 12, 16, 96 and 972 respectively. Chakras are closely linked to the endocrine, nervous and circulatory systems, but they do not belong to the physical body and cannot be seen with the naked eye.

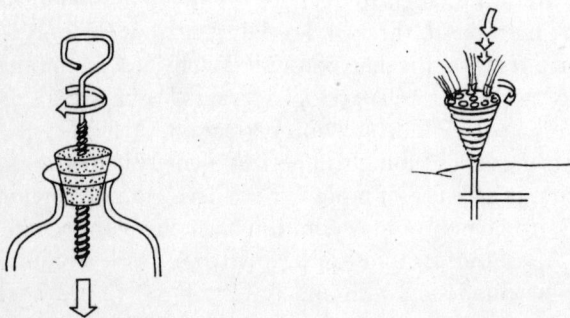

Fig. 2: *The spin of the chakras and the resulting flow of energy follow a rule similar to Maxwell's corkscrew rule of electromagnetism*

Maxwell's corkscrew rule of electromagnetism shows that if a right-handed corkscrew is imagined to be rotated so that the tip of the screw points in the direction of the current, the direction of the thumb's rotation shows the direction of magnetic lines of force. The movement of our chakras follows the same rule (Fig. 2). If you hold your four fingers around any of the chakras with your fingertips pointing clockwise (as an observer would see) then the thumb indicates an inward movement of the current. However, if you curl your fingers in such a way that their tips point anti-clockwise, the thumb will indicate the movement of current outwards. Thus, a chakra that rotates anti-clockwise is a 'closed' chakra—not conducive to the intake of energy.

Normally the chakras spin very fast, sucking the universal energy into our body and directing our hormonal secretions. However, as we grow older we develop negative patterns of thinking and living that slow down some or all of the chakras and sometimes even reverse their direction, causing an energy imbalance that results in various diseases and accelerates the ageing process. You can feel the influence of the chakras with the help of a pendulum, as it will start rotating on its own under the influence of any of the chakras when brought near that chakra's field.

Chakras are, again, the contact points where the *manomaya kosha* (mental body) integrates with and controls the *pranamaya kosha* (energy body). I lift my arm because the pranic energy from the *pranamaya kosha* follows a desire or thought from the *manomaya kosha*. The thought is like a radio wave; the chakras are like antennae. From the chakras, thought waves are passed on to the *nadis*—our body's electrical circuitry. For thought waves to flow in the circuitry of nadis, they need the pranic energy from the pranamaya kosha, much as a radio is supplied by batteries or electricity. Finally, the processed thought waves get transformed into perceptible movement in my arm, just as radio waves get transformed into sound waves at the speaker.

In everyone other than yogis, chakras and nadis work involuntarily, with no conscious intervention from the person. Yogis can, if they so desire, consciously use these chakras like step-up transformers to increase the pranic flow in the nadis.

Trying to suppress or deny particular emotions freely often results in blocks in the corresponding chakras—so do not hide your emotions from yourself, even if you decide for some reason to hide them from others. Reiki, pranic healing and chakra meditation are some of the ways to keep your chakras in youthful condition.

The seven energy vortices are located along the spine as shown (Fig. 3). Within each energy vortex are seven more vortices, each designed to transfer energy to the corresponding kosha. The seventh and first chakras are at the ends of the main vertical power current, which flows up and down between them and along the spine. The rest of the chakras are bipolar, funnel-shaped vortices with tips at the vertical power current. From these tips, each chakra extends about an inch, widening to a diameter of about six inches.

Each chakra emits energy according its own characteristics.

The root chakra (red), at the coccyx bone at the bottom of the spine, is associated with the adrenal glands. As the body's survival centre, it relates to issues of scarcity and abundance. A healthy root chakra supports a strong faith in life and will to live, and tunes us into the universe's abundance of food, money, shelter and health. This is also the repository of familial (immediate and extended), educational, racial, social and cultural information that gives each of us a unique identity. A blocked root chakra can lead to feelings of fear.

The second chakra (orange), or *hara*, located at the level of our sexual organs, corresponds to the spleen in men and the uterus in women. First impressions and nostalgic memories are stored here.

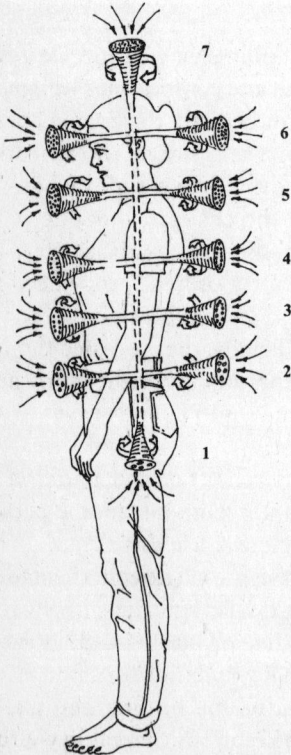

Fig. 3

Sexual attraction and creativity both stem from this chakra, and it is through this chakra that we receive and perceive *others'* emotions and sexual feelings. A diseased *hara* can cause fertililty issues and relationship problems. In women, this is also called the lower heart chakra.

The third chakra (yellow) is at the solar plexus, a man's power or control centre. Corresponding to the pancreas and liver, it is associated with digestion. It reflects a person's will, personal power, authority, self-control, physical and spiritual energy, and self-esteem. Issues related to alcoholism stem from a diseased solar-plexus chakra.

The fourth chakra (green), located in the centre of the chest near the heart, is associated with the heart and the thymus gland. This is the most important chakra for healing purposes. Through this chakra, we give and receive love, creating and strengthening cords to those with whom we are emotionally involved—family members, lovers, friends and so forth. A blocked heart chakra leads to apprehensions that others do not support us. The fourth chakra channels energy to the heart, circulation system, thymus gland, vagus nerve and upper back.

The fifth chakra (light blue), located at the bottom of the throat, corresponds to the thyroid and parathyroid glands, and is associated with communication, expression and creativity. When we find it difficult to express ourselves clearly or honestly, or to express our emotions at all, the throat chakra might need to be healed.

The sixth chakra (indigo), located in the centre of the forehead, relates to the pituitary gland. This chakra gives us intuition, paranormal perception or other psychic powers, and the ability to see the Latent Oneness.

The seventh chakra (violet or white), located just above the head, is associated with the pineal gland on the physical plane. Through this chakra we perceive spiritual guides and receive their guidance on our path to self-realization.

The important thing to note here is that constant use of Reiki over time helps heal the malfunctioning chakras. Once they are healed and balanced, not only our health but our very life is healed and balanced, too. Hence, Reiki is more than just a therapeutic tool—it is a way of life.

MODERN MEDICINE IS MISSING THE POINT

Modern allopathic medicine considers disease to be the result of the external environment, chance unfortunate happenings, genetic disposition, chemical imbalances or harmful eating habits. The focus is on the physical body only—the external sheath and its interaction with the physical world around it. The goal is to bring about chemical changes that provide relief, yet this relief is usually only temporary and even then is not without side effects.

The problem with this approach to health is that the micro-organisms that cause disease soon get acclimatized to the chemical scenario that follows the use of medicines and they adapt accordingly, resulting in a need for progressively more or stronger medication. This constantly shifting chemical scene starts affecting healthy organs as well as diseased ones—often with dangerous consequences. Often people die not because of their original disease but because of the havoc wreaked by the unhindered use of medicines. The solution is not to discontinue the use of medicines but to discontinue our obsession with and unnecessary dependence on them. Many of us have lost trust in the healing powers of Nature and our own bodies; we consider medicines a panacea. Instead of interpreting a headache as a message from the body and trying to understand it, many of us reach for a tablet without a second thought.

Antibiotics have proved a boon in the fight against many serious infections and diseases, so they deserve our respect and acceptance; but where is the justification for prescribing them for a cold or the flu virus? Thanks to propaganda from pharmaceutical companies, almost every nation on Earth spends billions of dollars and other scarce resources every year—not on *health* but on *mere temporary relief* from already-present diseases. This is akin to watering the leaves instead of the roots. Our short-cuts are cutting us short. Nature, however, has not built any short-cuts to health; it wants us to constantly learn and grow. Short-cuts deprive us of the invaluable opportunity to learn and grow from experience, especially illness. Every disease has a lesson for us, and if we evade the process of learning that lesson, health and happiness will continue to elude us.

Once health is understood as a manifestation of our inner state, a lion's share of the investment that organizations spend on getting temporary relief for their employees shall instead be spent on strengthening their subtler selves: training in positive thinking, yoga, proper diet, effective breathing, meditation techniques and so forth. The individual will then take full responsibility for his health, a shift in attitude that will improve his well-being and contain the unnecessary drain on our precious resources.

There is only one healing agency in this universe, and that is the healing energy of the latent oneness. Therapies provide a catalytic environment, but healing always comes from the same source—and this is what Reiki is. More and more medical doctors are realizing this, and moving towards holistic solutions.

We need not wait for those who are slow to change their paradigms. We are being ushered into a new era, and it is exciting indeed!

2

Reiki: A New Mystery

WHAT IS REIKI?

Reiki is a Japanese word made up of two roots: rei and ki. *Rei* means 'universal' or 'spiritual'. *Ki* is the Japanese equivalent of the Sanskrit *prana*, which means 'life energy force'. In fact, *ki* has an equivalent in almost every ancient language. The Polynesian Hunas knew it as *mana*, and in Hebrew it was called *ruach*. It is the *chi* of the Chinese, the *ka* of the Egyptians and the *baraka* of the Sufis. The Greeks called it *pneuma*, the Native American Iroquois *orenda*. More recently, Russian researchers have called it *bioplasmic energy*.

Rei combined with *ki* in Japanese, however (Fig. 4), means 'universal life energy force' or 'spiritual life energy force'—and *reiki* is more commonly understood as a simple hands-on healing system of incomparable ease and efficacy. Rediscovered by Dr Mikao Usui in Japan in the late nineteenth century, it can be used to heal oneself as well as others.

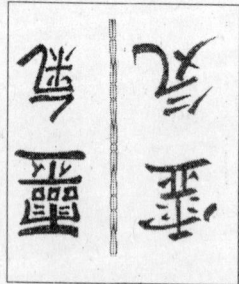

Fig. 4

Reiki is the primal energy. Philosophers, thinkers and mystics have taught us since time immemorial that *the universe is not made up of things, but of energy*. Modern physicists have now validated this belief of the great minds of all time—especially the ancient Eastern mystics—that the myriad forms the universe appears to take are nothing but energy impulses impregnated with information and pulsating at different frequencies. Reiki is, in fact, the fundamental energy of which the universe is made up. Reiki is therefore everywhere, and exists as everything. It is all-pervasive, and is unknowable yet can be experienced directly by anyone.

Reiki is a journey. It lets us retrace our steps through the blocks of forgetfulness that we create, however unintentionally, to keep ourselves from painful experience—and dissolves them in the process. In short, Reiki is a journey to rediscover our core essence through a reintegration of our being—a dissolving of walls to let parts reunite with the wholeness and oneness to which they once belonged.

Reiki energy is spiritual in nature. Correct practice of Reiki tends to correct any imbalance in the speed and direction of the spinning chakras, or energy vortices that provide an interface between our physical bodies and our auras (see 'The Secret Human Anatomy' in the Introduction). This process corrects any energy imbalance resulting from a disharmonious pattern of absorption and re-circulation of the cosmic energy within the human system—leading to all-around physical, mental, emotional, psychological and spiritual health. Reiki calms the mind and strengthens the user's life force. It reconnects us to our very core essence. This reestablishment of a connection with our core essence makes us realize that we indeed are unlimited; we have the power to manifest whatever we want for ourselves simply by intending to do so.

Reiki reestablishes our lost connection with the oneness that surrounds us in a multiplicity of forms. All human problems and diseases result from the illusion of separateness. The birth of Newtonian physics came in the wake of the Cartesian concept (named after René Descartes) of a world divided into spirit and matter. Newtonian physics was therefore divisive in perception, and gave us a mechanistic model of the world that dominated scientific thought until the beginning of the twentieth century.

If the divisive Cartesian world view and Newtonian physics resulted in the development of classical physics and technological advancement, it also broke down our wholesome attitude towards life into a fragmentary one, if only subconsciously. Inner fragmentation between the mind's will and the body's instincts has mirrored itself externally in the rise of men who see their fellow humans and the earth solely with the eyes of an exploiter. This epitomized the severance of man's links with his very roots—the Mother Earth.

The feeling of separateness makes us lonely and insecure, resulting in further delusions that world is imperfect and we need to transform it if it's going to take better care of us—an attitude that in turn gives rise to arrogance and conceit. Sometimes the search for security leads us to greed, an urge to hoard power, money or social status. Greed breeds further insecurity and fear—fear of failure to achieve, or failure to maintain what we do achieve. The means we employ to achieve all these things often run contrary to our own value systems, so guilt ensues. It is interesting to note here that some people hold value systems that make them feel guilty if they enjoy anything— money, luxuries, sex or whatever—forgetting that God is Himself a personification of joy, peace and bliss. When we are overwhelmed with insecurity, greed, fear and/or guilt, life becomes too heavy to carry on with.

Participants in a Reiki seminar often feel the re-establishment of their connection with the surrounding oneness very soon, and this feeling is mirrored in their attitude towards other participants as the seminar progresses: they smile more, feel more connected to each other and feel more love. The feeling is reinforced with each healing that they give to themselves or to others, and finally becomes a part of their life. The same can happen to a patient who is receiving frequent Reiki healing sessions.

Reiki is not given but drawn. It is drawn in proportion to one's subconscious intention, as it respects the recipient's freedom not only to believe or disbelieve but also to choose the extent to which he or she believes or disbelieves. It is this very freedom that originally allowed us to dissociate ourselves with the latent oneness, and now allows us to reestablish our lost connection with it.

Reiki can only be used for noble and positive ends—to heal. Reiki is nothing but unlimited and unconditional pure love-energy of the Latent Oneness for all that comprises it. This love-energy is the greatest vibration available to mankind. One of the most curious things about Reiki is that you can make no mistakes in its use—it has its own intelligence. The provider of Reiki energy is merely a channel. As Reiki is used more often, you will notice another curious thing in due time: Reiki starts suggesting things to you through your intuition.

Though it is impossible to use Reiki to cause anyone harm, Reiki may release suppressed negative emotions—anger, depression and so forth—against one's expectations. This is a natural part of the healing process, and contributes to personal growth. Reiki is not one's own energy; it simply flows through the channel's body, hence the practitioner does not feel depleted or weak after a session.

The flow of Reiki is the result of the intention of the channel. The channel moves *ki* or *prana* simply by placing his hands on the body to be healed, whether his own or someone else's. Reiki energy enters from the crown chakra from the north (in the northern hemisphere) or from the south (in the southern hemisphere), then moves through the forehead and throat chakra down to the heart chakra before flowing out through the channel's palms in a counter-clockwise helical path.

With regular use of Reiki, old mental and emotional blocks start dissolving. Reiki removes blocks that keep us from being in touch with our divinity, and prevents new blocks from forming. This dissolution of blocks also makes way for a progressively clearer, easier, more active channel through which a copious stream of Reiki energy can flow. With regular use of Reiki, creativity finds new wings, and divinity expresses itself in new ways. Lost balances within the body are reestablished; the body, mind and spirit begin to work in complete harmony for perhaps the first time. Joy replaces fear as our motivating force. We begin to stay calm, cheerful, happy, energetic and stress-free regardless of external happenings. With this kind of mental and emotional state, our body's resistance goes up, and it becomes virtually impossible for us to fall ill.

The process of dissolution of blocks within is mirrored in the dissolution of limitations without. People who use Reiki report that negative patterns in their lives seem to iron themselves out. For instance, some people find that just before they are going to reap the benefits of their efforts, someone else snatches away their due; others, in personal relationships, fear loving people because they have made foolish decisions in love before. Patterns such as these, which we usually dismiss as bad luck, begin dissolving with the dissolution of our mental and emotional blocks. However, it does take time and courage to come to terms with these fundamental changes.

Reiki is almost too simple and easy to be believed. One of the most difficult tasks I encounter in my life with Reiki is making people believe that something as simple as Reiki can bring about such profound changes in a person's life. Until people try it, they continue to have doubts, doubts and more doubts. Our rational mind and ego tend to come in the way of accepting the experiences of Reiki patients at face value. We tend to think we are intelligent and rational while those who report the miracles of Reiki are simplistic, gullible and lacking in scientific attitude. We forget that if we believe only in what is adduced by today's science, there would never be any progress in it. A shirt should be cut according to the body, not the body according to the shirt; similarly, our science should incorporate *all* our observations, including those that look irrational, and then search for the underlying reasons. To reject an observation simply because it cannot be explained or understood by contemporary science is intellectual dishonesty, and runs against the spirit of true scientific inquiry.

Reiki may not be visible to the naked eye, but it is as verifiable as any other invisible energy, and thus does not require blind faith. Our strong bias and conditioning in favour of what is material or tangible makes us assume that Reiki is merely wishful thinking, a mere belief or a kind of self-hypnosis, auto-suggestion, hypnotherapy, faith healing or placebo effect. Some think we are just imagining it, making it all up. Reiki is none of the above. Reiki's healing effects have been scientifically verified on plants and animals.

Moreover, Reiki is effective whether or not you believe in it. The only attitude required is a healthy attitude towards anything you know little about. Tell yourself, 'It might work or it might not work; I don't know. I am open to either possibility. Let me see what happens.' When you challenge Reiki by saying, 'It is unscientific. There is no reason for me to believe in it. I am sure it won't work. Let it prove otherwise,' you are not showing your loyalty to a scientific attitude; you are only revealing your bias against something before it has had a chance to prove itself to you. Such an attitude towards any exploration can hardly be called scientific. A truly scientific temperament does not jump to conclusions based on prejudice. You don't have to believe in an idea to be open to it. Being open simply means refusing to let our preconceived notions—whether favourable or unfavourable— interfere with it.

A beam of Reiki energy coming out of a person's palms is as real as electricity or magnetism. Kirlian photographs have shown a difference in the Reiki channel's hands before and during a healing session, leaving no scope for any doubts about Reiki being real. Here is a photograph (Fig. 5) of a Reiki master's hands before and after he started sending Reiki (distance Reiki, in this particular case). Both the sender and receiver of Reiki feel its flow in the form of varied but unmistakable sensations. Though most of us feel the flow of Reiki the first time we try, some people may require more sessions to sensitize themselves. Still, however, Reiki is effective whether we feel it or not.

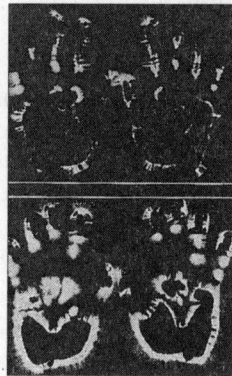

Fig. 5

Reiki requires energy exchange. Another difficult task I have encountered in my life with Reiki is to make people believe that losing their *hold* on something (money, for instance) will only ensure its easy flow back *into* their lives. I have seen people struggle for months and sometimes even years to decide whether they should spend money to learn something that is supposed to be spiritual in essence. They wonder whether someone who asks a fee can be a genuine teacher—because we have unconsciously nurtured a belief that a true teacher is free from greed, and that spiritual things are supposed to come free. They are supposed to come free because there are no takers for them; it is presumably the taker who is doing a favour to the giver by agreeing to receive them. This belief is nothing but our own arrogance, which we project on to the teacher as his greed.

No other energy-healing system can match the safety, simplicity and ease of Reiki. There have been many energy-healing therapies since time immemorial. What sets Reiki apart is the fact that no other system is as simple, effortless and easy as Reiki, both to acquire and to practice. Whereas other disciplines can take years of learning and practice, Reiki power can be acquired forever through an attunement over a weekend. Reiki attunements—mystic initiations or empowerments passed from the Reiki teacher to the initiate—empower the initiate to start healing him- or herself and others within a day's time. The attunement itself takes just ten to fifteen minutes.

Reiki acts and heals at the very roots of the problem—the energy body. Reiki does not heal the body or mind directly, but only steps up one's inner healing potential through one's energy body. This is one reason why Reiki works best when accompanied by healing at other levels, such as a cleansing and energizing diet, appropriate physical exercise, the release of bottled-up emotions, interpretation of the hidden messages an illness might be trying to convey. Revelations can then be followed up with the necessary change: mentally repeating powerful healing affirmations, visualizing that you have been cured (if you are ill) and developing an attitude of gratitude and respect towards your body,

Reiki is neither provided nor received through the conscious mind. Its effectiveness or efficiency does not depend on the conscious will or faith of the patient. It can neither be *pushed out* by the practitioner or *pulled in* by the patient's body through conscious will. Both practitioner and patient can, however, create optimal conditions for healing. A relaxing and peaceful environment, loose and comfortable clothes and a sense of complete trust and surrender to Reiki do facilitate a more effective flow of Reiki, and thus may result in a more effective healing process.

Reiki's popularity is growing at an exponential rate because of its ease, safety and efficacy. It has absolutely no prerequisites, as it does not depend on qualifications that can be learnt through a conscious mind; people from all walks of life are learning and practising it all over the world. Reiki's uses and applications are limited only by our own imaginations, which is why it is being acquired and practised by doctors, engineers, healing practitioners, masseurs, physical therapists, psychologists, students, housewives, executives, corporate leaders, people who are interested in personal growth and self-realization and people who are simply curious.

WHAT KEEPS PEOPLE FROM GIVING THEMSELVES THE GIFT OF REIKI?

If you believe only in what you see, then you are limited to what is on the surface.

—Wayne Dyer

The history of the world has shown that people are slow in accepting those truths that are beyond the human senses. At an unconscious level we are heavily biased against intangibles; we are conditioned to believe in only those things we can perceive directly. To do otherwise is to accept being seen as uneducated or illogical, and our egos cannot afford this. However, history has proved time and again that when people dare to transcend their prejudice against intangibles, they often bring humanity to a new milestone. For example, a great revolution in the field of medicine came with the findings of Louis Pasteur that infection, putrefaction and disease were caused by organisms too small to be seen with the naked eye. People were slow to accept such a concept when it surfaced, but the eventual paradigm shift sparked a chain of discoveries and inventions that have totally transformed the world of medicine.

Today, when science is fast catching up with the timeless truths discovered by our *rishis* and sages, we are on the verge of coming to know and believe (like the medical scientists of Pasteur's time who struggled to come to terms with his findings) that the diseases, accidents, misfortunes, failures, emotional pain and misery in our lives are the results of chain reactions triggered by our own impure thoughts, perceptions, beliefs and attitudes. We can protect and fortify our destinies by 'pasteurizing' our thoughts, attitudes and behaviour through an inner integration of our being. Reiki is a journey towards this inner integration.

We tend to believe in new ideas more readily once they are acknowledged and accepted by an authority, or by the majority of the people around us. Only a few among us dare to hold beliefs that run contrary to those held by the majority. By extension, we readily believe something if we are told that it has been scientifically proven, because we take science to be an authority.

For an aborigine to disbelieve what can be accomplished through a cell phone or a remote-control device for a television set is only too natural. He may even hesitate to consider such a possibility, not because he is less intelligent or backward than we are, but because he is yet to experience the working of such an instrument. Twenty years ago you too would have behaved like him with the same skepticism if you were to be asked to consider such a proposition.

In the late 1960s there were no takers for the patent of quartz watches because the dominant Swiss manufacturers were trying to look into the future through the rear-view mirror. They found it hard to believe that watches could work, and in fact work better, without the usual springs, gears and bearings. Obviously they were blinded by their own perceptions of how watches should work; their successful past blocked their vision of the successful future. The Japanese, however, considered the new reality, dispelled the clouds of doubt in their mind and jumped over to the sunny side of the trench, leaving the Swiss manufacturers within their own prison of certainty. Japan, a country that had never had a presence in the watch market, emerged after 1968 as the new world leader in manufacturing quartz watches, and continues to lead the field today. Switzerland, which had dominated the watch market for almost a hundred years, had to relieve 50,000 of its 65,000 workers from the industry, and within ten years fell to hold less than ten per cent of the world market share.

Modern medicine stands today at a similar crossroads. Though an increasing number of people are realizing this and opting for holistic solutions like Reiki, a vast majority of people are still stuck, like the Swiss, in their own arrogance and rigid views. They find it difficult to believe that healing can work, and sometimes work better, than the usual scans, blood tests and medicines. Their successful past blocks their vision of the successful future.

Disbelief often says more about the person carrying it than about the concept in question. We tend to accept only what is least challenging to our existing beliefs, however limiting and stifling for our spirit this may be. We do not use everything we have, but rather what we know, believe and *remember* that we have. Learning to use something regularly comes by habit or constant repetition.

People may dismiss Reiki by saying:

1. Reiki sounds too good to be true. In addition to our bias towards the tangible, we are taught from childhood that nothing is both good and easy in this world. Yet Reiki is both. Of course, it is effective only if practised. It is indeed not very effective unless you commit to its five principles and make time for it regularly.

2. Reiki is a money-making gimmick, a fraud. We often take the world to be full of charlatans and frauds, but the world is also full of honest, sincere, dedicated and committed people. A true Reiki teacher or channel never tries to convince you to undertake Reiki against your wishes; he only clarifies Reiki if you have doubts. He never makes promises. He never claims to have healed anybody, and admits openly that it is not he but Reiki that heals. Being a mere channel of Reiki, not a healer himself, he cannot guarantee any cure on Reiki's behalf. He will only point out that whatever Reiki does is in the best interest of everyone. He does not keep you in the dark about his fee, or energy exchange, and does not bring down his rate to compete with other practitioners. A true Reiki teacher has no competitors; he sees other practitioners as part of the same mission, respects them sincerely and may even recommend them if he himself is busy or inconveniently located. A true Reiki master works *with* but never *for* money. His money may come *through* you but not *from* you.

Charlatans exist in every field, and Reiki may not be an exception. All imperfections are a part of the universe's perfection. Some of us *want* to cheat ourselves, however unconsciously, so the universe arranges charlatans to facilitate what we want. After discovering the fraud, we can either look within, realize our mistake and learn from it, or we can blame others for our bad luck and invite similar other frauds, one after the other. You will not encounter frauds if your intentions are pure.

If you ever think you have reason to doubt, doubt the person, not Reiki. Before doubting either, get conversant with the essentials of Reiki and the conditions under which it works. And, of course, remember that Reiki is not a substitute for professional medical advice, especially in emergencies or in the case of serious terminal disease. Reiki should be used only as a supplementary therapy in such cases.

People have a tendency to play it safe. They would rather not lose what they have come to acquire (money) than exchange it for something intangible. They do not realize that money has no intrinsic value; it is only worth something when used to acquire what the buyer needs or wants. In India, people have only just begun to spend money for the good of their spiritual selves, but the number is increasing day by day.

3. Reiki is against my religion. Some people assume Reiki to be a kind of religion, and think that the pursuit of Reiki constitutes insincerity towards their own religion. I have heard of the heads of religious sects directing their followers not to use Reiki, though without citing any reasons. Religious people are daily misguided against Reiki by sect leaders who have no knowledge of Reiki, indeed nothing but misperceptions, myths, prejudices and preconceived notions—and in some cases fear and insecurity—on which to base their advice.

Some people treat life the way they treat their television sets. With a remote control in their hands, they keep changing the channel, always worried that there might be a better show elsewhere. They lack faith in their decisions, and the patience to stick to something; they sow a seed and remove the soil every five minutes to check whether the seed is sprouting. Similarly, they keep seeking advice until they find someone who gives them the advice they want to hear.

Reiki is simply a healing therapy involving spiritual energy, It is not a religion, nor is it <u>*against*</u> *any religion or belief system.* It is only *for* all that is in harmony with Nature and the Latent Oneness. You do not need to change or give up your religious beliefs or lifestyle to use Reiki; in fact, Reiki may enhance your religious convictions.

4. Reiki is an inferior alternative to modern medicine, with no scientific basis. An open and scientific mind is humble; it accepts that it does not know everything, even in the fields it already knows best. Reiki works. Whether or not you reap its benefits does not depend on whether its scientific basis has been discovered or not. Even today we don't know everything about light and electricity, but we use them because they work. Reiki's scientific basis has yet to be determined, and it shall be determined one day. But the evidence that Reiki works is so commonplace today that scientific proof of its efficacy is immaterial.

In an experiment conducted by Dr Janet Quinn (assistant director of nursing at the University of South Carolina) at St. Vincent's Medical Center in New York, recipients of Reiki healing were found to have significantly enhanced immune functions (CD4 to CD8 ratio). In an experiment conducted by Wendy Weztel at Sonoma State University, blood samples taken before and after first-degree attunements revealed enhanced haemoglobin (the part of the red blood cell that carries oxygen) and haematocrit levels (the ratio of red blood cells to total blood volume), and a reduction of undesirable substances such as cholesterol. Another experiment found that the blood pressure of participants in a Reiki I seminar tended towards normalization—those suffering from high blood pressure experienced a reduction in blood pressure and vice versa. In California, Dr Daniel Wirth of Healing Sciences International in Orinda, California, discovered an acceleration in the healing process after human wounds were subjected to a few minutes of Reiki treatment. Similar experiments with mice and plants have revealed faster healing of wounds and improved growth and enhanced production of chlorophyll respectively.

As mentioned above, Reiki is not an alternative to modern medicine and should not be promoted as such. Rather, it is a tool to harmonize the physical and the energy bodies. Because it acts at the causal level of disease, it must be used only to *supplement* professional medical help, especially in serious cases. While modern medicine is disease-oriented, Reiki is health-oriented—it focuses on restoring and maintaining health rather than fighting disease. It does not think of removing darkness; it just switches on the lights.

5. Material things can be influenced only with material things. Chemicals in medicine act upon those in the body to bring about change, but how can chemicals be influenced by energy coming out through someone's hands? People have been taught that disease is a chemical state of the body which will remain as such until acted upon by medicine or surgery. Material things or chemicals are only forms of energy vibrating at a particular frequency that happens to be slower than those of heat, light or electricity. Matter is a secondary manifestation of the fundamental energy of which this universe is made up. Not only can energy affect matter, but it does so all around us every day. Electricity is energy; it acts upon machinery all over the world. Sunlight can burn a piece of paper when focused through a convex lens. The invisible energy waves emanating from a remote control influence the distant television set.

Moreover, we already know that thought energy can affect our bodies. Thoughts of extreme fear can make us sweat, or make our stomach churn, or make the hair on our skin stand up. Many of the changes that take place in our physical body during the various stages of sexual intercourse are driven by thought energy. In photosynthesis—the process by which plants make their own food—the green leaves of plants absorb sunlight in a pigment called chlorophyll, then combine the light energy with carbon dioxide and water to produce sugar and other chemicals. And so on.

6. I am already healthy and happy. No one is healthy enough on this planet. Everyone needs healing. Health and healing are ongoing processes. Will you be happy on your deathbed that you lived the kind of life you are living now? Will you be able to say with all honesty that you have done all you could have done for others, loved them enough, spent enough time with them, made a difference to those less privileged than you?

When I got my first spectacles, I realized all I had been missing. The world grew suddenly clearer and more vivid. The same can be true for those of us who think they are healthy enough not to need healing. Health is not the size of your biceps or an absence of any serious ailment; health is your ability to feel the oneness beneath the apparent multiplicity of forms, and it is your ability to identify, believe and live your dreams.

7. I am too busy. It is not enough to be busy; it is more important to ask what you are busy *doing*. We all are seeking happiness, and many of us spend every moment on this quest, but most of us are still unhappy. Look at the four quadrants below and you will see why this is so: we tend to short-circuit our route to happiness. For example, when we smoke we focus on the instant pleasure we derive from it, not on the distant sorrow we invite.

II	I
Instant Pleasure / Distant Pleasure (Quadrant to be expanded)	Instant Pain / Distant Pleasure (Quadrant wherein to spend most of your time)
· Reiki · Showing that we love and care · Meditating · Listening to soothing music · Learning about self / Improving our knowledge	· Exercising · Learning · Responding to negative acts with positive acts (Forgiving)
III	IV
Instant Pleasure / Distant Pain (Quadrant to be avoided)	Instant Pain / Distant Pain (Quadrant to be eliminated)
· Eating fried food and junk food · Taking revenge · Smoking and drinking · Making decisions based on short-term gains	· Misusing our power to hurt others · Expressing our anger · Worrying about things that cannot be helped · Feeling guilty without learning lessons for the future · Planning revenge

The recipe for happiness is to spend the maximum portion of your day (or life!) in Quadrant I, spend more time in II, less time in III and no time whatsoever in IV. When you spend maximum time in QI you expand the spectrum of activities that will ultimately be enjoyable for you, even if you find them a bit of a pain right now. Over time, you can increase your liking of a particular beneficial activity (that you currently feel repelled by) by simply doing it more often, so that your brain grows more familiar with it. By doing so, you slowly change activities that you do not like to do but are beneficial (Q1) into those that provide both instant as well as distant pleasure (QII).

Similarly, whenever you spend time in Q3, focus on the distant harm the activity causes, rather than the pleasure of the moment. Envision how it will harm you, and realize how it will mercilessly dissolve your dreams and goals.

So now, when you say you are busy, don't forget to inquire which quadrant you are spending time in. Learn more about Reiki through this book, and then decide whether you are still too busy to make time for it.

Note: The activities that give instant pleasure and instant pain can differ from person to person. Some of the activities that fall in Q1 for some may fall in QII for others and vice versa. Quadrant IV, which inflicts both instant and distant pain, may seem counter-intuitive, but we have absorbed the vain hope that these painful things might bring us distant pleasure.

8. Reiki is too slow. Results take too long. This is a common complaint today. We seem to have lost the capacity to relax or be patient; we want instant results. This is one reason for all the discontent and frustration around us. As you bring Reiki from Q1 to QII, you will not regret that it's slow; once you start enjoying it, you will want it to be even slower. You will develop the ability to relax and be patient with everything, and you will start loving yourself more for that. The results of Reiki healing are not always delayed; they depend on various factors, including openness on the part of the patient to receive Reiki and take responsibility for his or her ailment (including giving up the habits or responses that incurred disease in the first place). Acute cases heal very quickly, whereas chronic conditions do take longer.

Reiki is far wiser than we are. It knows what to heal first and what to take up later, in the best interests of the healee. For example, Reiki may decide to repair a particular organ before repairing the one the healee is more concerned about. It may even start healing diseases that have not yet been diagnosed. A man who wanted to give up smoking did not think he was benefiting from Reiki, but he started developing an interest in tennis. Soon he was playing very well, and he wanted to play even better but his lack of stamina got in the way. Finally he decided to quit smoking of his own accord. So trust the route Reiki is taking to accomplish complete healing within you.

9. Reiki is boring. I don't like to sit still. Some people think they are too active to feel comfortable with this kind of therapy. Try listening to your favourite music—the soothing kind—while you provide or receive a Reiki treatment. Try doing Reiki while watching TV or, when you are starting out, even talking to a friend. Remind yourself that you deserve to relax, and Reiki is a natural way to do so.

10. This 'miraculous healing' is mere coincidence. Yes, even if the benefits of healing are favourable coincidences and not the direct effects of Reiki, they are still brought out by Reiki. People encounter such 'coincidences' more often once they come in contact with Reiki. Reiki may bring about precisely the combination of coincidences to set your life right.

11. I oppose guru worship. Reiki does not advocate guru worship, unlike many religious sects. A guru is one who has mastered his senses, whereas the term *Reiki master* simply indicates someone who has acquired the qualification to hold Reiki seminars and conduct Reiki attunements. A Reiki master does not demand worship; he is more like a friend who equates you with himself and respects the fact that you are as divine as he.

I have personally found that deep gratitude for one's Reiki teacher does help one's progress in Reiki. You may feel differently, but in any case you should avoid criticizing your Reiki teacher or talking about him in derogatory terms, as he does represent the most sacred Reiki energy.

12. Reiki is too embarrassing. Friends and colleagues will ridicule

me. **My family might object.** I myself have relatives who might be laughing at me behind my back. It is natural on their part to do so, and with all the humility at my command and all my love and respect for them, I must simply ignore what they feel about me or Reiki in this regard.

In many areas of life, you have two alternatives. You can slow down your learning process and spiritual evolution so as to become one with the masses, who move at a languid pace for fear of being ridiculed, or you can give up caring for those who ridicule you and go on to respect your own evolutionary needs. Everyone has a unique frame of reference. Like you and me, our relatives and friends are moving towards one goal just as all rivers are moving towards the same ocean. Our paths may be different, but the path for every river is the perfect one for it.

13. Reiki will interfere with the working-out of my karmas. Nature's purpose in introducing and maintaining the karmic principle in the universe is not to seek revenge or some kind of universal justice. Nature does not seek to punish you; it only seeks to educate you, to move you through your spiritual evolution. The purpose of any disease or discomfort is to teach us a particular lesson. When you offer to learn honestly what a particular discomfort wants to teach you, you obviate the necessity for that discomfort to remain. It will serve no purpose thereafter, and will thus leave you and seek the next student. You do not work out your karma only by going through hardships; you work it out better and more easily by offering to learn the intended lessons. Reiki healing is holistic and integrated—it seeks to teach you while healing your physical and energy bodies. So in this respect, Reiki does not interfere but actually facilitates the working-out of karmas.

14. I will lose my personality. No—Reiki will only fine-tune your personality to bring out the best in you. The best in you is the real, unique you.

15. Such powers come only from demons or Satan. I don't want

to join with them to play against God. If you ever find yourself doubting the truth or spirituality of a particular entity, consider its effects on you. A good way to check the authenticity of a rose is to watch the honeybees—they never hover over an artificial rose, no matter how exquisite it looks. Ask yourself whether you feel a pull for Reiki within your heart. Be sure you address your question to your heart, not to your mind or ego; the latter can have artificial or cosmetic reasons for feeling a pull towards anything. Many of us cannot even distinguish between the two. Once you focus on your heart chakra and address this question to your emotional self, you will feel the pull towards Reiki in your heart: it will fill your heart with love and beauty, give your mind peace and contentment and let your soul regain its purity and bliss, effects only God or His representatives can bring about.

16. There might be serious side effects that aren't known yet. A new allopathic drug may have side effects that emerge as an unpleasant surprise late in the process; allopathic drugs are *artificially created,* so time alone can tell whether or not they are in harmony with nature. In contrast, the side effects of things holy in nature are never unknown or unpredictable. Unholy agencies never hesitate to harm others or take revenge, but like God or any true representative of His, Reiki can never bring harm. It can only bring love, harmony, abundance, beauty, contentment and peace wherever and whenever it is used. 'If God is for us, who can be against us?'

17. I tried Reiki. It didn't work. Unlike hypnosis, auto-suggestion, faith healing or the placebo effect, Reiki is not a psychological phenomenon. Reiki flows from the hands even if the *channel* does not believe in it, and certainly flows into the receiver's body, wherever required, in spite of his disbelief. The only exception is the rare case in which the receiver's real intention is not to explore Reiki but to disprove it. For some people, belief in disbelief is too precious; something like Reiki can threaten the collapse of the very edifice of their (dis)beliefs.

Indeed such people may create a strong enough mental or emotional block to impede the flow of Reiki, if not prevent it altogether. Reiki does not demand blind faith, but Reiki *is* pure love, and love cannot exist without a sense of freedom at its foundation. So consider whether you were open enough to the idea that the phenomenon of Reiki is real.

Moreover, sometimes the receiver does not feel Reiki even when it is actually working, and bringing about the required healing in the body. Reiki often takes a healing route quite different from the one we expect or favour. In its unquestionable wisdom, Reiki always works in our best interests and may have other plans for us.

18. I tried Reiki, and the pain actually got worse. I turned to my doctor for help just in time. Different people respond differently to Reiki. Aggravation of symptoms, known as physical chemicalization or a healing crisis, is a common phenomenon. It occurs because a large amount of energy is being drawn, so one possible effect is the 'clustering' of the toxins to be dealt with. Though naturally unpleasant, this is a favourable sign that your body is responding to Reiki. The symptoms will dissipate quickly with further treatment, in the next two or three sessions.

The phenomenon is best understood through the analogy of cleaning a used ink bottle. As you pour water in it and flush it out, the water that comes out is extremely inky. The second time you fill and flush out the water, it will still be dirty, but less so. You repeat the process until the water that comes out is as clean as the water you pour in it.

In the case of chronic conditions, the aggravation may repeat itself after a few weeks, when Reiki moves into the second cycle of cleansing. Again, the intensity of symptoms decreases with every new cycle. The last cycles can be the most difficult or time-consuming, as at that point Reiki is attempting to drive out the most stubborn blocks or toxins.

In some cases, pain or discomfort may be experienced even by those who had no symptoms prior to starting Reiki. This happens because Reiki can act upon and start attempting to heal a disease that has hitherto been lying dormant in the energy body, not having manifested itself on the physical plane just yet. Reiki often accelerates the mobilization of healing energy when it encounters an ailment, and this is experienced as pain or discomfort.

19. I am already on medication. Reiki can be combined with any therapy, such as allopathy, homeopathy, naturopathy, ayurveda, acupressure, shiatsu or rolfing . Reiki does not require you to stop any ongoing medication or treatment pertaining to other therapies. As Reiki raises your life-energy force, it will only accelerate the healing process and make the medication more effective.

20. I am too unspiritual a person. This kind of therapy won't work for me. Reiki works for everyone. It does not depend on your feelings or ideas about your being spiritual, intelligent and deserving (or not), nor does it depend on any previous experiences or notions about your learning abilities Each one of us is divine; we all have the same physical and spiritual anatomy. Once you are attuned, Reiki works, and works always in your best interests—provided you use it. The more you use it, the better it will work for you.

21. How can you heal me without diagnosing me? Reiki is holistic healing. It does not need to diagnose. All diseases are the result of some kind of imbalance in the body, and imbalance in any one part of the body affects the rest of the body as well. No part of the body can function in isolation. This is why a Reiki practitioner begins with a full-body treatment, whatever your ailments may be, and continues for at least four sessions, preferably more. During these sessions, he may come to know which organs are drawing more energy or need more energy, and may then decide to spend more time on those parts of the body. If time is very tight and the ailment is minor, a Reiki practitioner may think of attending only to specific parts of the body. If you already have a diagnosis, the findings of the Reiki practitioner may confirm it; alternately, Reiki's wisdom may decide to heal other areas first, if they are the underlying cause of the diagnosed disease.

22. I suspect something fishy—why does the master ask people to close their eyes during attunement? Why can't the secrets of attunement be shared? Since you will only be initiated into Reiki once in your life, it is best to feel the great harmonizing process taking place within you during the attunements. Keeping your eyes closed helps you do precisely this. It also allows you to feel the appropriate gratitude for this gift you have given yourself— a desirable state during the attunement process. Attunements are conducted by the master alone and do not need any active participation from the one being attuned; you need only cooperate and let the master do his work with full concentration. Keeping your eyes open, or half open, or trying to steal a glimpse of what the master is doing will only distract him and keep you from feeling what is happening within you. Moreover, even if you are able to see what the master is doing, you will not understand it, and it may unnecessarily keep you guessing the effects of each of his movements. In sum, keeping your eyes closed helps both you and the master discharge your respective roles appropriately.

23. I cannot make the drastic changes required to try this therapy. Reiki does not demand any drastic changes in your lifestyle. However, for twenty-one days after any attunement you are indeed supposed to abstain from tea, coffee, non-vegetarian food, eggs, cigarettes and alcohol because they put unnecessary strain on the body when it is undergoing a thorough cleansing operation. You are also supposed to minister self-healing to all points of the body during every one of these twenty-one days. After that you can resume your normal lifestyle, with no changes except to set aside some time for self-healing or healing others at your own convenience.

24. My friend tried Reiki, and it seemed to work initially, but he no longer feels any charge in his hands. He has discontinued it. Reiki attunements are irreversible, and once acquired Reiki cannot be lost, even if you don't use it for decades. Not feeling the charge does not mean Reiki is not flowing; Reiki is drawn by the healee in proportion to his openness or need at that particular part of the body. One does not always 'feel' the flow of Reiki.

25. I don't want to remove my clothes or have the practitioner touch my body, especially a person of the opposite sex. You do not need to remove your clothes for Reiki. I think this misperception comes from the sketches in some Reiki books, which show the human body in the nude. Such sketches have been used in some books only to clarify the Reiki hand positions, and the books often include a note to this effect. If you do not want the practitioner to touch you anywhere, simply tell him so, and he will keep his hands an inch from your body at all times. If the practitioner is advanced (Reiki II or above), he may even provide you with distant healing, for which it is not necessary for you to be physically present, though it is recommended that you appear for at least the first four sessions. Reiki practitioners are themselves very conscious, and they take care as a matter of course to keep their hands an inch from the body while giving Reiki on or near the breasts or private parts. Reiki can pass through not only clothes but plaster casts, blankets, wood and steel, hence Reiki may actually hasten the healing process on parts of the body covered with a cast.

26. My disease is chronic, so it may be too entrenched for Reiki to be of any help. All chronic diseases can benefit from Reiki. Normally patients are already undergoing treatment from a qualified medical practitioner, in which case Reiki can accelerate the healing process by releasing blocks and toxins from the body. The time to a cure depends how old the disease is, how committed and open you are to the healing and how detached you are from the results, even after doing all that you are supposed to do as a good patient. Acute diseases, on the other hand, are of more recent origin and higher intensity. In these cases you should see a qualified physician first, and if the pain is intolerably acute you should rush to a hospital for professional medical help. Reiki does not always result in quick healing as it fixes problems holistically, which can take time.

27. Infections need antibiotics. Yes, you may feel relief much faster with antibiotics, but avoid indiscriminate and excessive use thereof. As long as you are not too uncomfortable, let Reiki heal you, or at least let it support the medication prescribed by the qualified medical professional.

28. My last Reiki teacher claimed big things that (not surprisingly) he could not prove. It may be that Reiki was not interested in proving anything to you against your wishes. Reiki respects your freedom to disbelieve it, and may not wish to proceed it if it does not find you open and receptive. Beware, however, of those who promise big things—this is contrary to the spirit of Reiki healing. Such people might be immature, or they might be outright charlatans. A true Reiki practitioner is humble; he knows that the healing comes through Reiki alone, and that Reiki is too sacred to be turned into propaganda. Reiki alone knows whether the patient's expectations will match the outcome.

Apart from causing a great deal of misunderstanding, those who promise big things give Reiki a bad name. The famous saying that it is better to have an intelligent foe than a foolish friend is very much true for Reiki. If you cannot befriend Reiki, you won't be harming Reiki much, but if you befriend Reiki without using your wisdom, you will be doing it a great disservice.

29. Why haven't I heard of Reiki before? We normally do not attract anything into our lives till we are prepared for it and feel a need for it. For this very reason, we don't hear anything about said phenomenon until such time. If you are busy grappling with other things that appear important to you, Nature may not feel like throwing something valuable in front of you, as you will be disinclined to value it. The very fact that you are reading this book shows that at a conscious, unconscious or karmic level you have been desiring and preparing yourself for Reiki.

30. I am too lazy to stick to it. Laziness does not come from lack of energy; it comes from lack of belief in oneself. And lack of belief in oneself results from lack of self-knowledge. Self-knowledge comes when we start making a concerted effort to search for our lost spiritual identity. Reiki can help you in this reintegration. Just make a start, and you will see door after door open up to usher you into a world beyond your wildest dreams. God is only waiting for you to say a big 'yes' with all your heart. The moment you commit yourself, Providence will move, too.

We tend to remember things only when we consider them important. For most of us, nothing is important except a secure, easy and predictable life with good health, lots of money and very smooth and slow changes. We take little or no responsibility for changing ourselves; we want everything without having to pay any price. We resist change until it becomes inevitable. But a new horizon of possibilities is open to all those who are ready to know, believe and remember to learn Reiki and then use it constantly. Every day, all over the world, millions of people are coming under the Reiki umbrella, experiencing silent revolutions in their personal and professional lives, enriching themselves with all-around physical, mental, emotional and spiritual health, improved creativity and intuition, better relationships, a deeper sense of security and a growing trust in their sense of purpose and the meaning of life.

31. I have a better alternative. There are many paths; Reiki is not the only one. Do, however, check the conviction of your statement. Does it come from your ego or your heart? If it does not come from your heart, you may need to review your belief.

If you are deeply satisfied with your all-around growth as a result of what you are following, then I can only congratulate you and ask that you write to me. I am eager to hear about it. I have tried many self-transformation tools and have not found anything more effective or easier than Reiki.

32. Warmth is natural to the human body—what does Reiki have to do with it? If extra warmth is all I need, I'd rather just use a warm-water bottle. No, no, no . . . you are getting it all wrong. Reiki is not just body warmth; warmth is only one sensation through which many people experience Reiki energy. There are many others; indeed, Reiki is sometimes experienced as ice-cold water pouring in. Moreover the warmth experienced with Reiki is distinct—it often gets too hot to be confused with body warmth. Try placing the hands of someone who is not a Reiki channel in the same place where you experience warmth under a Reiki channel's hand, and see whether you feel just the same. It is not the warmth that heals.

33. Can someone give me a live demonstration? Ask a few people who have tried Reiki. You may not experience anything dramatic in the short space of ten to fifteen minutes, especially if you are not open or receptive to it.

THE EFFECTS OF REIKI

Reiki works on physical, mental, emotional and spiritual levels by restoring the lost balance between the mind, body and spirit. Because it transcends both time and space, it can even affect events beyond time and space. Reiki also heals one's karma. Diseases originate in the energy body; Reiki heals any rips and tears in this body and strengthens it. Reiki heals at the causal level of disease, and thus eliminates the effects. Clairvoyants who can see auras have confirmed a marked difference in the quality and strength of the aura of any participant before and after a Reiki attunement.

Reiki soothes pain, hastens the healing process, stops

bleeding (if not too profuse), relaxes and rejuvenates the body, balances the chakras and energy body and balances the two hemispheres of the brain. The recipient's breathing rate, heart rate and pulse rate all slow down, bringing deep and complete relaxation. Some patients drift right off into slumber during Reiki sessions.

Some people report a flowering of intuition or the development of psychic abilities. Though Reiki affects different people differently according to their needs, it commonly:

- Induces deep relaxation
- Releases toxins
- Dissolves blockages
- Supplies healing energy
- Steps up the body's vibrational frequency

Possibilities with Reiki

- Reiki enhances your ability to respond to life situations more appropriately without stress. The ability to keep your cool and cheer regardless of external circumstances leads to increased self-confidence and trust in the Latent Oneness. You stop 'sleepwalking' through life; you become more and more 'awake'. Lessons meant to be learned from life situations are grasped more easily, obviating the necessity for harsher routes to learning them.
- Reiki can transform life situations, transcend time to affect both the past and the future, and therefore heal both past karma and future events.
- Reiki can help manifest your desires or intentions, if they are in harmony with the common good of all.
- Reiki can be used to heal the environment and Mother Earth. For example, scientists can use it to heal the ozone layer, and it can be used to heal inanimate objects (since, strictly speaking, there are no inanimate objects; objects that seem so are only grosser manifestations of the same cosmic energy) and make gadgets function better and last longer.

- Reiki can be used in industry for better production, safe and harmonious operation, improved synergy and cohesion among workers, improved customer relations, better use of resources, improved creativity, reduction in waste and increased sales.
- Reiki can help develop intuition, which in turn can be used to find creative solutions and to invent and improve gadgets.
- Above all, Reiki can be used to make the earth a cleaner, greener and more loving, peaceful and blissful place to live.

Advantages of Reiki

- Reiki is simple, quick and easy to learn and use.
- Reiki can be done anywhere and anytime. You do not need any special space or equipment; all you need is a pair of hands and the right intention. You can perform Reiki on yourself while queuing in a shop, waiting in an airport or railway station, commuting, talking to others on the phone or even in person, watching television, or waiting for your boss to go through a file or take a phone call. You can be sitting, lying or standing.
- You can even use Reiki in your office. Since Reiki develops a deep trust in the oneness and perfection of the universe, all negative feelings and unnecessary politics come to a grinding halt. You start seeing that whatever happens is in your best interests, and that all the energy people waste trying to prove themselves is for naught. Once you realize this, your own energy is gradually redirected towards more positive pursuits. Customer satisfaction is nourished by your genuine love for your colleagues and external customers. Accidents, waste and hurdles are drastically reduced when there is harmony in the environment. One friend of mine, a senior officer in the blast furnace of a steel plant, has found that whenever there is a mechanical breakdown, he can use Reiki to set things in order. A very senior officer with Indian Railways, much to his pleasant surprise, managed to strike a good rapport with some otherwise hostile union leaders

through the use of Reiki. I am sure there are thousands of professionals all over the world who already use Reiki to achieve maximum efficiency, harmony, success and general perfection in their workplace. [1]

- Great benefits can accrue after as little as one Reiki session. Reiki cannot replace modern medicine, but it often accomplishes what medicine cannot, with minimal discomfort and expenditure.

- Reiki helps your body eliminate harmful micro-organisms before they affect your health. Dormant and forgotten capabilities start surfacing, and you find yourself feeling more and more creative. The learning process accelerates, and you intuitively find new applications for what you are learning.

- Reiki helps replace the energy lost in the process of healing from surgery or allopathic treatments such as chemotherapy. After any operation or intensive treatment the body needs to readjust, and badly needs energy to grow new tissues, fight germs and so forth.

- Reiki retards the aging process and improves alertness and mental potential.

- Reiki can help dissolve surgical scars, if applied within two years of the operation.

- Reiki attunements last a lifetime, and perhaps longer.

- Reiki can be used to heal your pets, plants, children and friends as well as yourself.

- Reiki is completely safe, as the intake is controlled by Reiki's own intelligence according to the needs of the healee. For example, if the healee has a headache that stems from a digestive problem, Reiki will direct itself to the digestive system even if the healer's hands are still on the head.

- The practitioner also receives healing while giving it to the healee. In other therapies, the practitioner can feel drained after the treatment.

---

1. The author is a pioneer in coaching organizations on how to harness the powers of Reiki to enhance corporate performance and achieve desired results.

Limitations of Reiki

■ Successful treatment depends on the receptivity of the healee. If the healee is not receptive or open to Reiki, he may not be able to draw Reiki in desirable amounts, and thus may not be healed quickly. If you are subconsciously (or even consciously) convinced that you deserve illness because of your sins, you are likely to close all doors to recovery.

■ No one consciously wants to be ill, but at a subconscious level one might see some benefits in illness, as it absolves one of some daily responsibilties. Illness can also draw attention, affection, sympathy and love from others, which can be more important than physical health. In such cases Reiki may not be entirely effective, as Reiki respects one's right to *decide* to be ill.

■ Reiki cannot be a substitute for direct life experience; it cannot teach all the necessary lessons for self-growth. One needs to watch one's responses from moment to moment to develop sensitivity.

■ Serious illnesses or emergencies requiring immediate relief, such as profuse bleeding, should be dealt with immediately by a medical professional.

FINDING A GENUINE REIKI MASTER

Anyone can become a Reiki channel (healee) over a weekend. Reiki is not achieved; it is acquired. It cannot be self-taught through books, exercises or meditation. The only way to acquire Reiki is to be initiated by a bona-fide Reiki master.

To find one, simply look for the nearest Reiki master in your locality and gather more information about it and find out whether he or she can book you into the next seminar. Look for newspaper advertisements, look under 'Reiki' in the telephone directory and search the internet. You can also purchase any book on Reiki and seek the help of the author (myself obviously included) in locating the most appropriate master for you. If you would like to be treated individually and already have a first-hand feel for Reiki, you can make an appointment for a purely 'healing session' as well.

Reiki is, unfortunately, becoming a generic term. People are adding all kinds of prefixes to the word. Moreover, of course, there is the faint chance of falling into the trap of one who is not a genuine Reiki master. I have only heard of one such case, but it pained me. A teacher is known to some extent by his or her students, so you must make inquiries with the students of the master you are considering.

I strongly believe that one gets the teacher one deserves. Sometimes, instead of a teacher, we are actually looking for someone who can tell us how great we are, or how great we were in our past lives. And that's exactly what we get—someone who who is looking for students who will readily pay just to be flattered. Such students and teachers are made for each other, and they find each other. The first step towards ensuring that you get the right teacher is to ensure that your intentions are genuine—devoid of any desire for ego gratification, of any doubts about the preciousness of Reiki and hence of any hesitation to pay the price the teacher asks.

Make sure you have the time and intention to commit to Reiki. It is futile to try to learn Reiki if you do not make the time for it. I would estimate that more than ninety per cent of those who learn Reiki I give it up within the first three months. Some are not able to complete the twenty-one-day post-attunement regimen. Among the ten per cent who do not give up, only a few practise Reiki every day, even though there could be hardly anything easier in this world. *Reiki is effective only if practised. It is ineffective without your commitment.* No false hopes, please! Ask yourself exactly why you intend to learn Reiki.

Some people are not sure whether learning Reiki can be worth so much money, and try to play it safe by looking for a teacher who will charge peanuts; and they get precisely that kind of teacher. Reiki is often done *with money* but should never be done *for money*. A Reiki master with pure intentions may charge a fee for healing sessions and attunement seminars, but his or her deepest intention is to heal you at all levels of your being, and thereby to make you grow spiritually and enable you to to do the same for others.

A genuine Reiki master:

- will not bargain for the fee to rope you in. Under exceptional circumstances, he might bring down the fee at his or her discretion.
- shows love and respect towards other Reiki masters; does not appear to be in competition with them. Will not mind referring you to a Reiki master closer to your home.
- involves himself in healings, too.
- issues signed certificates to participants on completion of the seminar.
- knows his Reiki lineage and talks about his masters with love and respect.

To make a decision:

- Visit one or two of your prospective Reiki master's seminars as a guest. Sit relaxed, take a few deep breaths and try to feel with your heart. Do you feel a pull towards this person? Do you feel easy and comfortable accepting him or her as your master? If so, he or she is probably the one meant for you.
- Ask yourself if you can genuinely respect the master you are considering. This is important, because how much you learn from him or her depends upon the extent of your surrender and trust. If the bond of love and respect between the two of you is weak, you are likely to discontinue the training or carry on with it half-heartedly, which obviously will deprive you of Reiki's full effects.

It is quite perfect for each one of us to be imperfect; our imperfections are part of the universe's perfection. Even if you find some slight imperfection in your master's personality, it is important for you to accept him or her as a human being. Remember that he, too, is on an ongoing spiritual journey.

ATTUNEMENTS

One thing that sets Reiki apart from other energy healing systems is the fact that the empowerment of Reiki is *not achieved* but *acquired*. The secret spiritual ritual through which it is acquired is known as an attunement. Attunements allow us to re-link ourselves to our forgotten, limitless self by dissolving the self-created blocks that keep us from it. These blocks are the results not only of what we hold back in this life, but also of what we have held back in previous lives. In fact, attunements do not give the recipient anything new; they simply open and align us to what has been there but been forgotten.

The attunement is not a healing session, though attunements do bring about profound healing at various levels of being. The purpose of an attunement is, rather, to make one a *channel* of healing energy so that one can use Reiki to heal oneself and others. Attunements are conducted in a calm, sacred environment by a bona fide Reiki master only. The one to be initiated sits calmly with eyes closed throughout the attunement process, which takes around ten or fifteen minutes.

The methodology of attunement is supposed to be kept secret by the Reiki master and revealed only to those who are committed, serious enough and spiritually ready. Secrecy is maintained only to ensure that those who are not qualified to conduct attunements do not attempt to do so, and thus to keep the channels' trust in Reiki intact. Those of us without proper experience do not understand the subtlety involved and may unnecessarily invite karmic repercussions. Moreover, attunement is a sacred process; there should be no scope for amateurs to fiddle around with it. The purity and strength of the empowerment to pass on attunements is a sacred flame that has been handed down from one master to another since the time of Dr Mikao Usui. A bona fide Reiki master who is physically present can personally watch, guide and fine-tune his student's progress, unlike those who offer written, postal or Internet Reiki attunements.

Different people feel and experience attunements in different ways. Some see colours, lights, religious symbols (such as a cross, om or lingam), or a past-life experience; others feel warmth or peace; some feel almost nothing. A few may feel nauseous soon after the attunement; this happens because of the immediate release of certain blocks and toxins, and signifies that whatever negativity the person was holding has been released. Ironically, nausea is thus a welcome event. Through attunement the Reiki master passes energy to the initiate in an amplified state, resulting in the creation of a channel for Reiki—it can enter from the crown chakra and move through the next three chakras before leaving through the minor chakras in the palms.

Attunements trigger a twenty-one-day cleansing process. During this period the recipient's body adjusts and re-adjusts to the changes taking place at all levels of his being. It takes an average of three days for *each* of the seven chakras to adjust to the stepped-up energy levels. Because the body gets busy releasing its accumulated toxins, healees often report temporary surges of anger, greed and lust on an emotional level and symptoms such as loose motions and runny nose on a physical level. A few people may even experience reddish-brown urine. Healees must drink lots of water to facilitate the body's ongoing detoxification, rather than try any new medication. Though each healee undergoes profound changes at all levels of being during this twenty-one-day period, not everyone feels change at a conscious level.

No one knows for sure how and why attunements work. Reiki cannot be understood by logic, for logic is based on past knowledge, which in turn is based on perceptions received through our senses—whereas Reiki involves forces and agencies that cannot be perceived directly by our senses. Whenever I begin my lecture for a seminar, I pray to these forces and agencies to bless me with their presence and guidance during the whole seminar. With indescribable gratitude, I have often received and felt a blissful magnetic charge all around my being as their immediate acknowledgement and response to this prayer.

Sometimes the feeling is so intense that my throat gets choked with emotions and I feel like crying like a child. The miracle of attunements must be experienced to be believed; it cannot be described. Those who have experienced it, especially those who carry on with Reiki, know it to be a life-transforming event.

First-degree attunements act mainly on the first kosha, which relates to the physical body, facilitating metabolization of increased life-force energy. The first-degree initiation involves four attunements designed to step up the vibration rates of the heart, throat, third-eye and crown chakras. Each attunement affects these chakras only indirectly, however, as it acts at a level beyond that of the chakras, i.e., at the very core level. In fact, as a result of these attunements, there are corresponding re-adjustments in the lower three chakras too. The final step 'seals' the channel in the open state, so the recipient is now able to channel Reiki energy for the rest of his or her life.

The second-degree attunement (there is only one) activates the three second-degree symbols that can be used for distant healing, and focuses on purification at the level of the etheric body. This brings about healing on the emotional, mental and psychological levels. The twenty-one-day cleansing these particular attunements trigger relates mainly to the emotional and mental levels. Many unresolved emotions, unhealed past-life situations and negative patterns come to the surface in order to be healed during the next six months or so. The initiate may or may not feel comfortable with these changes, and may or may not recognize the inherent opportunity to free him- or herself by attempting to heal these old patterns. The third-eye chakra is greatly affected, resulting in improved intuition, which may also result in the gift of psychic abilities for some and enhanced inspiration for self-realization for others. There is a corresponding stimulating effect on the root chakra.

During the twenty-one days after your second-degree attunement, you may experience lower-back pain or enhanced sexual urges. This may be due to activation of the hara chakra, the seat of Kundalini. With the help of the following energy-circulation exercise, you can, if you wish, transform this energy to a higher chakra instead of using it for sexual intercourse:

- Lie on your back with your eyes closed, knees raised and touching, feet slightly apart and hands at your sides with the palms up.
- Take twelve breaths, imagining that there is a black and white sphere the size of a tennis ball within your head (Fig.6).
- Take another twelve breaths, visualizing your genitals to be dark blue.
- Take another twelve breaths, visualizing the occipital lobe of your brain as dark blue (Fig. 7).

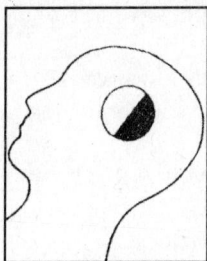

Fig. 6

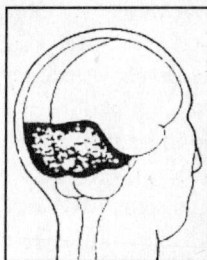

Fig. 7

The third-degree attunement activates the master symbol (symbols will be discussed shortly), which enhances Reiki's power by a factor of eight. At this stage the post-attunement twenty-one-day period affects the spiritual body more than the physical body, so most recipients do not feel any symptoms at all, though some do feel the need for more rest and sleep.

Like second-degree Reiki, third-degree Reiki involves only one attunement that enhances the channel's capacity to transmit energy. Clairvoyants and scientists working on human energy fields have both confirmed that Reiki attunements expand, purify and intensify one's energy field. And, of course, the more you use Reiki, the more efficient an energy channel you become.

Methods of attunement can differ from master to master, and some who claim to have tried almost all of them confirm that all of them work. It is not the methods or rituals alone that work; it is the grace of Reiki.

There are times when channels do not feel Reiki flowing

through their hands and start assuming this is because of their own sins or spiritual misconduct. Reiki behooves us not to judge people; we must accept people as they are even if we do not approve of their actions. That being so, how could Reiki judge *you*? Reiki is pure unconditional love of the Latent Oneness. It will never forsake you, even though it gives you the freedom to choose not to use it for any reason.

If you find yourself feeling that Reiki is not flowing through your hands, it is probably for one of the following reasons:

1. Being newly attuned to Reiki, you have yet to develop sensitivity to Reiki's subtle flow.
2. Your level of sensitivity is temporarily low because of a hectic daytime schedule. Reiki is flowing; your body just needs a little more time to relax.
3. Reiki is indeed not flowing through your hands because Reiki is not sent—it is received. You may be trying to *provide* Reiki and finding your body unreceptive because of an energy block or because Reiki is simply not required in that particular place.

REIKI SEMINARS: WHAT TO EXPECT

You can become an effective Reiki channel and use Reiki to heal yourself and others soon after the first level of attunement. The first, second and third levels of attunement qualify you as a first-, second- or third-degree Reiki channel. Some masters even give both levels of attunements on the same day, while others (like me) insist that you spend a few months practising Reiki I before moving on to Reiki II, as you need this time to understand, adapt to and assimilate the changes the attunements bring. However, third-degree attunements are given only at the invitation of your master.

If, after you acquire the three degrees of attunement, your master feels it is appropriate, he or she may invite you to learn the secrets of conducting the attunement process yourself. In this case the teacher will also train you in conducting seminars independently, which may involve watching and assisting him or her in his or her own seminars. Only when your teacher is fully satisfied that you can conduct your own seminars will you be issued a certificate permitting you to do so. Some call this level of achievement the fourth degree; others call it the III-B degree; and others integrate it with the third degree itself.

The golden rule is not to rush. Give yourself a little romance with Reiki before you proceed to marry it. Reiki III and masterships are serious things, and one should go in for them only if you are serious enough to dedicate your life to teaching Reiki. Do not think in terms of making Reiki a means of livelihood; such a mindset indicates lack of preparation for the life of a Reiki teacher. As in any profession, the pressure of earning money can make you compromise on certain essentials. You might hasten a participant to higher levels of attunement, for example, even when her evolutionary needs demand more practice with the lower degrees.

First-Degree Reiki Seminars

Simply put, the first level of Reiki enables you to heal yourself and others through touch. Many of the Reiki miracle stories that we hear or read about are brought about through Reiki I only.

In a first-degree Reiki seminar you will learn what Reiki is, how Reiki affects and benefits us (and how it doesn't), Reiki's history, the five principles and other introductory matters. After this general lecture, you will learn the various points on the body where Reiki is drawn, and which hand positions facilitate the process. Some masters ask participants to put their hands in some of these positions to feel the sensations there, if any, before the attunement so they can clearly feel the difference afterwards. You will then perform one exercise designed to emphasize the importance of gratitude, and then you will be called one by one to the attunement room. After attunement, participants share their feelings and experiences thus far. Lunch is served.

The afternoon session begins with Nada Brahma, an exercise

meant to remove various blocks in the body to facilitate the flow of Reiki through its newly laid channel. After a brief session in which, again, participants share their experiences, you will have another lesson in hand positions. The group is then divided into pairs, and participants take turns providing Reiki to one another under the observation and guidance of the master.

Though it is not important to feel warmth or other sensations associated with Reiki, most people feel something in the very first instance, doing either self-Reiki or partner Reiki. Others may take two or three days to get sensitized. As Reiki is a very subtle energy, it usually takes some time to get fully tuned to it and appreciate it fully. Often the seminar ends with a Reiki circle or ring, in which participants sit silently in a circle, holding the hands of those on either side of them, and feel the flow of Reiki energy. Finally, the master distributes certificates, gives some general tips and reminds you to be regular in your Reiki practice.

First-degree Reiki healing (not attunements) can be provided to plants, pets, crystals and gadgets—all living *and* non-living things. Animals can be treated as humans are; animals' organs are located at similar positions in the body. Reiki can be given to the full body or, if the animal is small, behind the ears. The length of the session depends upon the animal; it will let you know when to finish the session by simply going away when it has its fill. In the case of an aquarium, simply place your hands on the walls, which in turn will charge the water. Reiki can also be given to the water and food you consume (see 'Reiki and Diet' in Chapter 3), as well as whatever medicines you might be taking.

The euphoria and enthusiasm that follow the newly acquired Reiki I often make one impatient to acquire Reiki II as soon as possible. A genuine Reiki master will ask you to practice Reiki I sincerely for another twenty-one days, and preferably for a month or two, before thinking of Reiki II. Remember that 'Reiki I' and 'Reiki II' are merely labels unless you practise them; you should be more concerned about growing with Reiki than about collecting labels.

Benefits of Reiki I:

1. Reiki I enables you to draw Reiki, let Reiki flow through your hands and provide Reiki wherever healing is required. You do not need to concentrate, change your lifestyle, meditate or do any breathing or other exercises. Reiki is there whenever you wish it to be so. However, as a mark of gratitude, it is proper on our part to express this wish as a simple prayer to Reiki.

2. Reiki protects the channel from passing his or her own energy to the client or taking on disharmonious energies from him or her, so disharmonious energies are not spread.

3. As a result of the opening of the heart chakra, which enables you to see the reflection of the same source in everything, you will start developing a natural love for everybody and for all that is. Every time we engage ourselves in healing, Reiki takes the same route through the heart, which in turn absorbs a bit of it. Of course, this change comes in proportion to the extent to which you are open to it.

4. Reiki I brings to the surface parts of your life that have not yet been integrated, including any unresolved issues. Personal growth is not served on a platter; the decision to address such issues is yours.

5. Reiki I helps you develop a sense of responsibility towards your life, a desire to take it into your own hands.

6. You develop trust in the underlying sacred oneness that nourishes and nurtures all of us, and hence you begin to accept, love and respect all forms of life. The illusion of separations slowly starts fading, and you learn to go with the flow of life instead of resisting it.

7. You develop intuition and sensitivity for the energy field all around you.

Second-Degree Reiki Seminars

Reiki II provides still more powerful tools for self-growth and healing, since it enhances our potential at all levels of our being.

In a second-degree Reiki seminar you learn some powerful symbols, and these are firmly anchored in your aura during the attunement—after which Reiki flows through the channel more intensely and efficiently. The symbols may vary slightly from one master to the next, but in any case they are not supposed to be shared with the uninitiated (including Reiki I practitioners), so I will not reproduce them here.

Reiki II has all the benefits of Reiki I but is far more powerful: you can provide or receive it long-distance. With practice, you can even exchange information with your absent companion in addition to providing Reiki. The spread can be thousands of miles; Reiki does not become fainter or weaker with distance. All you need is the person's name, photograph or description. You can send Reiki to several people in the same place or in different places; you can even 'programme' Reiki to reach a person at a particular time for a particular duration. You can send Reiki to a particular place, country or even the whole earth. (To enhance the effect, groups can send Reiki together to Mother Earth or to a country.) You can energize precious stones with Reiki before you wear them. Reiki II enhances awareness and sensitivity, and helps heal negative emotions, karmic patterns and mental disorders. It can be used to cleanse rooms of their negative energy.

Once you learn second-degree Reiki, your sessions will become shorter and more effective. Providing yourself or anyone else full-body Reiki might take just twenty minutes, for example, whereas in Reiki I it might have taken almost ninety. Charging your food before each meal will facilitate assimilation and reduce the effects of any harmful substances in the food.

Through second-degree Reiki we can learn direct contact with our own subconscious, or with the cosmic mind. Apart from the physical self, Reiki II can heal and harmonize our emotional and mental selves (kosha 2 and kosha 3). Though the content and presentation of the seminar vary from master to master, the basic approach remains the same. Usually a Reiki II seminar begins with participants sharing their experiences of Reiki I and clarifying any doubts they have about Reiki I or

Reiki in general. You are then taught the three symbols and asked to spend some time drawing them, which may take half an hour or so. Then, as in a Reiki I seminar, the participants are called one by one for attunement to second-degree Reiki. After attunement, you have a hands-on session of self-Reiki and then provide and receive full-body Reiki with a partner using the newly acquired symbols.

Though I do not give their names and drawings here as a mark of my respect for their sacredness, the three symbols are known as:

1. Mental/emotional healing symbol. All diseases originate at the mental or emotional level as some kind of imbalance in the energy body. By dissolving blockages on the emotional and mental levels, this symbol establishes harmony within one's being. Apart from negative emotions and attitudes, it can also be used to treat addictions. For example, if you are in the habit of eating too much, write, 'Eating well for healthy weight control', draw the symbol next to it and administer Reiki to it every day for fifteen to twenty minutes. You will find that the need to overeat will dissolve. This process re-establishes the lost balance and coordination between the left and right hemispheres of the brain. Regular and prolonged use of this symbol can enhance memory and awaken extra-sensory and intuitive powers.

2. Distant or absentee healing symbol. The purpose of this symbol is to bring energy down into the heart chakra and open the mind so that Reiki can operate beyond space and time—it connects the heart chakras of the channel and the healee through an invisible energy conduit. The symbol seems to streamline the diverging beams of Reiki energy (akin to ordinary light waves) into laser-like parallel beams, and thus allow them to flow easily without dissipation of intensity. This is how the limitations of distance are transcended. The symbol is also used to heal past-life traumas or future events that you want to be successful (say, an interview or a seminar). All this can be difficult for the uninitiated to believe and comprehend; if you find it so, ask a Reiki II channel to send you Reiki from a distance so you can see the truth for yourself.

3. Power symbol. This symbol steps up the power of Reiki, and acts as a catalyst and activator. It also envelops an object or client in a shield of white light, which fends off any harmful influences. Hence this symbol is used as a power-enhancer at the beginning of treatment and a protective shield towards the end.

The above symbols come from the Japanese *kanji* (script) or Japanese language. The names of the first and third symbols are Japanese, but the script is not purely Japanese. The second symbol is entirely Japanese in origin. The symbols are like keys that establish contact between you and the supreme power without bringing you to an altered state of consciousness. Because they are sacred, the symbols should be drawn accurately and recited mentally with full devotion and respect. (It helps if you learn to draw them small.) Every healing with symbols should be finished by drawing and mentally reciting all three symbols in order, with deep gratitude for each one. Finally, express your feelings in a mental prayer, which might run like this: 'With the love and mercy of Reiki, I declare [whatever you mean to heal] healed complete and whole. I am grateful to you, O Reiki. Thy will, O Reiki, be done.'

Benefits of Reiki II:

Programming Reiki

You can use this technique to provide Reiki to a person or event when you cannot be physically present. Write down the date, time, event or person's name requiring Reiki, and then write the intended outcome. Imagine a laser-like beam of white light shooting out of your heart chakra and your palms and enveloping this paper completely. Draw the three symbols in order on this cloud of light, which has gathered all around this paper carrying your intention. Then spend fifteen minutes (or whatever time you can spare) repeating the power symbol, chanting its name thrice every time you draw it. Draw all three symbols once more, and then declare that the event or person is receiving Reiki at the intended date and time. Visualize, with complete trust, this taking place.

Alternately, you may choose to give Reiki to your visualization of the intended outcome while a calendar and clock in the background show the requisite date and time.

Healing the Past and Future

Do you ever repent not having acted as you should have at some point in the past? Do you ever regret the day when, under the influence of friends, you took to some undesirable habit that has taken its toll on you ever since? Don't you often wish you could travel back in time and change everything by reacting to events in a wiser way? Often an unfortunate incident in our formative years gets embedded in our being and becomes a source of constant disharmony, getting us stuck in negativity. If this is the case with you, Reiki offers you the opportunity to go back to that time and heal that situation now. Through Reiki, you can establish contact with the person you were at that juncture, heal the undesirable event and thus the consequences that entailed. This will free you of karmic ill effects and clear any obstacles to your growth. Of course, all this is possible only if you consciously admit and confess your wrong and promise sincerely to learn from your mistake.

Similarly, Reiki can be sent to the future. Are you anticipating a difficult time ahead? Perhaps tomorrow or the week after, you will attend a meeting that means a lot to you, and you are crossing your fingers in the hope that everything turns out well. Perhaps tomorrow the union leaders are coming for a tough negotiation. You know stress is not good for you, but you find it difficult not to worry. If you face such a situation now, try sending Reiki ahead to that moment.

For either the past or the future, the procedure is similar to that used for 'programming' Reiki. Imagine yourself in the situation to be healed, then imagine—in detail—things working out the way you want them to: the distinct colours, the sounds, the applause, the compliments, the joy, the happiness and all the rest. Shoot out a laser-like beam of purple or white light from your heart chakra, and let it gather around and envelop your mental picture like a cloud. Draw the symbols on it, one by one, reciting the name of each one thrice after you draw it.

Intention Reiki

Visualize the fulfilling of your intention in full detail, including your feelings. Send Reiki to this picture as described above, with or without a time frame as the case may be. (Actually, 'programming' Reiki is only a specific form of 'intention' Reiki in which we want to specify the date and time.) Whereas Intention Reiki may need to be sent every day for fifteen minutes or so till fulfillment takes place, 'programming' Reiki need only be done once.

Intention Reiki can be used to fulfil any of your intentions, which may range from healing relationships (that may or may not involve you), getting a promotion or a particular contract, financial growth, a successful seminar, conference or meeting, success in a competition or an interview, recalling a forgotten piece of important information, the health and long life of an appliance, creating the future of your dream—all that limits you is your own imagination.

When you cannot be physically available in a situation of general disaster, you can send Reiki to victims of famine, war, earthquakes, hurricanes, floods and accidents.

Reiki Box

Write down all your intentions precisely and briefly. These can include fulfilling your desires, wishes and goals, healing a person or event, giving up some bad habits and so forth. Now take a sheet of white A4 paper and draw horizontal lines with a pencil, an inch-and-a-half apart. Take a pen and copy each of your intentions neatly in one of the rows. Feel each intention deeply in your heart as you write it down. Now, after photocopying the paper for reference, cut the paper into strips along the horizontal lines. Collect the strips into a pack, roll the pack into a cylinder and slip it into a small box like the one that comes with photo film.

Give Reiki to this box twice a day for fifteen minutes, using the procedure described above: the attitude of gratitude . . . white light . . . a cloud of white light enveloping the box . . . Reiki symbols . . . repeat the power symbol . . . close with the three symbols, and declare with the permission of Reiki that your intentions have been healed complete and whole.

Giving Up Undesirable Habits

Picture yourself involved in your bad habit. Then imagine this picture to be slowly receding far into the distance, getting progressively smaller and hazier. Say to yourself that you are willing to release the inner need for this bad habit. Now imagine a new 'you' who happens to be free from this habit, practising the corresponding desirable habit and looking back from a distance at the undesirable habit of the past. Send a beam of white light from your heart chakra, and let a cloud of white light gather and envelop this picture. Send Reiki through symbols.

The procedure is the same if the undesirable habit is not yours but someone else's; just visualize that person instead of you.

Healing Dead People

Visualise the dead person alive. Send a white beam of light and pray for Reiki to flow. Cover the cloud of white light with the Reiki symbols. Say whatever you wanted to but could not say before this person died. Ask for forgiveness or forgive, as the case may be. Now visualize the person as satisfied, contented, cheerful, happy and peaceful. Declare him or her (or your relationship with him or her) healed, whole and complete. Close with the three symbols and white light.

Healing Gemstones

Exposure to sunlight and regular cleansing with water may not cleanse your gemstones of disharmonious influences. Providing Reiki with symbols reawakens the stones' lost powers. Again, follow the procedure described above.

Healing Tensions

Write down or declare out loud your worry or source of tension. Picture dissolution of your worries, fears, apprehensions and tensions. Send white light and the Reiki symbols.

Healing Blocks

Lie on your back with both hands on your hara chakra (an inch-and-a-half below your navel). Ask Reiki to guide you in identifying what is holding you back and why. Alternately, imagine a wall representing blocks or withholds wherever they may be in your body, and then imagine this wall and the corresponding 'withholds' and fears dissolving. Feel your enhanced energy and strength.

Distance Healing: Short Method

Repeat your chosen affirmations (see Chapter 4) to bring yourself into an attitude of gratitude.

- Hold the photograph of the person to be healed in your hand, and look at it very carefully. Close your eyes and try to internalize the photograph; focus your mind's eye on it completely. Imagine the person to be happy, joyous, cheerful, hale and hearty, smiling and completely healthy.
- Mentally write the person's name, or imagine it written beneath the photograph. If you can picture the person without the photograph, fine.
- Shoot out the love beam of white light and let it strike and envelop the entire mental picture of the healee. You are seeing only white light, but you are aware of the picture behind the light. Draw the three Reiki symbols in order, now repeating the name of the symbol thrice each time.
- If you happen to know that a particular part of the person's body is diseased, visualize it and focus your attention on it.

Imagine Reiki reaching it, and imagine yourself drawing symbols on it. Imagine that part of the body to be healthy now.

■ Provide Reiki for ten to fifteen minutes. See the patient as happy, healthy and peaceful. Close with the three symbols. Mentally thank Reiki and the patient.

Distance Healing: Long Method

■ Get into the attitude of gratitude.
■ Declare your body to be that of the patient.
■ Give yourself full-body Reiki. With every new hand position, declare that organ or body part to be that of the healee.
■ Close with the three symbols and the declaration that the body of the healee (say the name of the patient) is now healed complete and whole, and is yours again (say your name).
■ Mentally say, 'I am grateful to you, O Reiki. Thy will be done.'

Healing the Chakras

■ Sit cross-legged facing your partner, with your knees touching his or hers. Hold one another's hands. Look into one another's eyes and be with each other mentally, emotionally and spiritually.
■ Close your eyes for the rest of the exercise.

Focus your mental attention on your partner's crown chakra—deep violet in colour, with its tip at the centre of the crown. The crown chakra, an inch-and-a-half above the head, is your partner's link with the Latent Oneness of the universe, the sacred self. It is at this level one holds one's core beliefs, which may or may not be in harmony with the universal laws. Cover the chakra with white light and energy and provide Reiki as usual with the three symbols. See your partner's crown chakra being healed, bringing your partner a spiritual awakening. Visualize your partner's core beliefs being aligned with the universal laws. Declare your partner's crown chakra healed complete and whole.

Shift your attention to your partner's third-eye chakra—

dark blue and bipolar, with its tip on the centre of the horizontal axis passing through the third eye (a little above the eyebrows). The front part of the chakra deals with comprehension; the back part deals with step-by-step implementation of ideas. This is also the centre of intuitive powers and inner wisdom. Cover the chakra with white light and energy, and provide Reiki with the three symbols. Visualize your partner's third-eye chakra being healed and awakened, with enhanced intuitive powers and inner wisdom. Declare your partner's third-eye chakra healed complete and whole.

- Switch to the throat chakra—light blue and bipolar, with its tip at the third cervical vertebra (C3). This chakra is the source of energy for the thyroid gland, the bronchi and lungs and the alimentary canal; proper hearing, tasting and smelling faculties depend on the health of this chakra. The throat chakra is related to self-expression: the speaking of one's truth and the openness with which we give to and receive from others. Cover the chakra with white light and energy, and provide Reiki with the three symbols. See your partner's throat chakra being healed and awakened, resulting in a flowering of the ability to express him- or herself with clarity and with the courage of inner wisdom. Declare your partner's throat chakra healed complete and whole.

- Move to your partner's heart chakra—bright light-green and bipolar, with its tip at the fifth thoracic vertebra (T5). This chakra is the source of energy for the thymus gland, heart, upper back, vagus nerve and circulatory system. This front part of the chakra is related to love, the back part to will; a healthy heart chakra keeps the two properly balanced. Cover the chakra with white light and energy, and provide Reiki with the three symbols. Visualize your partner's heart chakra being healed and activated and imagine him bathed in the pink light of love, experiencing the resulting surge of feelings of uninhibited motherly love and compassion for all. Declare your partner's heart chakra healed complete and whole.

- Move now to the solar-plexus chakra—bright yellow and

bipolar, with its tip at the junction of the twelfth thoracic vertebra (T12) and the first lumbar vertebra (corresponding to the notch on the front of the torso where the bottom few ribs meet). This chakra is the source of energy for the pancreas, liver, gall bladder, spleen and nervous system; it relates to wisdom, strength and our ways of perceiving and relating to the world around us. Cover the chakra with white light and energy, and provide Reiki with the three symbols. Visualize your partner's solar-plexus chakra being healed and activated, and experience his or her blossoming of inner strength and wisdom. Declare your partner's solar-plexus chakra healed complete and whole.

- The next chakra is the hara—bright orange in colour and bipolar, with its tip at the centre of the sacrum. This chakra is the source of sexual energy and a strong immune system; a healthy hara relates to inner peace and stabilty. Cover the chakra with white light and energy, and provide Reiki with the three symbols. Visualize your partner's hara chakra being healed and activated, and see peace and a sense of stability descend on to your partner. Declare your partner's hara chakra healed complete and whole.

- Come now to the root chakra—red in colour and monopolar, with its tip at the intersection of the axis of the torso and the perineum between the legs. It is through this chakra that we get a sense of position and movement of the body in relation to other things. Here is the energy source for the adrenal gland, kidneys and spinal column. A healthy root chakra relates to physical vitality, a strong will to live, the trust that one will always get what one wants or what is best for one and that there is no scarcity of anything that one wants in this world. Cover the chakra with white light and energy, and provide Reiki with the three symbols. Visualize your partner's root chakra being healed and activated, and experience the resulting shift in his or her attitude from a sense of scarcity to a sense of abundance. Imagine your partner feeling totally secure and prosperous, beyond all wants. Declare your partner's root chakra healed complete and whole.

- To conclude, envision all your partner's chakras as totally overhauled—clean, glowing and spinning in a clockwise direction at the optimal speed. Imagine your partner surrounded by an abundance of success, abundance of prosperity, abundance of love, abundance of fame, abundance of beauty, abundance of happiness and complete fulfillment of his intentions, wants and desires. Declare your partner complete and perfect in every sense. Spend some time in this state, then slowly open your senses and gradually become aware of the room you are in.

Healing Plants and Animals

- While seeds only need about two or three minutes, room plants may need around ten minutes of Reiki. Bigger plants require second-degree Reiki.
- You may choose to give Reiki to the water itself (two minutes for each quart) before sprinkling it into the soil.
- Give Reiki to roots by placing your hands around the pot. Reiki helps newly potted plants to adapt to new soil with ease.
- Reiki may help stave off pests. Giving Reiki to pest-infected plants helps them develop resistance to parasites. Even if the pests drop away after treatment, you should continue Reiki for another four to five days, washing the leaves before each session.
- Giving Reiki to trees can be a rewarding experience for the peace and blessings they may shower upon you. Some Reiki channels claim to have received useful intuitive suggestions during this process.
- Pets can be given direct or distant Reiki (the latter is best if the animal is ferocious), as can the food or water they consume. Animals often turn the side or body part towards you where they feel the need for Reiki; watch carefully and be sensitive to their needs.

Healing Mother Earth

Take a small globe between your hands and declare it the real Mother Earth. Shoot out white light from your heart chakra and the centre of your palms, so as to engulf it all around. Start drawing symbols on the cloud of white light surrounding the globe, saying the name of each symbol thrice as you finish drawing it. When you come to the power symbol, go on repeating it for the next ten to fifteen minutes. (For better results, you may choose to repeat both the mental symbol and the power symbol.) You can also heal Mother Earth in a group of Reiki II (or Reiki III) channels. If you don't have a globe, simply imagine the earth or hold a tennis ball and imagine Mother Earth to have shrunk between your hands.

Reiki can be sent to great teachers and masters such as Lord Krishna, Christ, Guru Nanak, Lord Buddha, Lord Rama, Dr Mikao Usui, Dr Hayashi, Madam Takata, Paramhamsa Yogananda, Jiddu Krishnamurti, Shri Sri Ravi Shankar, your own Reiki master or anyone else you hold as a spiritual mentor. When you do so, Reiki reflects back on you with stepped-up power and intensity.

Needless to say, despite the excitement of being able to heal people from a distance, we should still do so only when asked, and only with the appropriate energy exchange. (Exceptions might be your parents, children, spouse, Mother Earth and the universe.) Despite the fact that Reiki II is stronger than Reiki I, its efficacy still depends on the receiver's attitude—on whether or not he wants Reiki and in what measure.

Third-Degree Reiki Seminars

Traditional Reiki teaches that Reiki III should be given only to those who are serious enough on the path of Reiki to want to make Reiki their life. The third-degree attunement is therefore not given on request; it is given by invitation only to those who are ready. There are no hard-and-fast rules, but normally you must spend more than a year practising Reiki II before your master will invite you on to Reiki III. More time and regular use of Reiki at each level enables you not only to enrich your own experience but also to assimilate the subtle developments taking place at all levels of your being. All this will prove useful if you become a teacher yourself, as you will then be called upon to explain to your students the correct way to use symbols—not to mention answer their questions and doubts—and you will not be able to do this if you lack personal experience and the spiritual maturity that builds up only slowly with regular use of Reiki. A Reiki master usually sits in meditation to seek guidance on whether or not to grant someone Reiki III initiation, so it is indeed an honour to be asked to serve Reiki in this degree.

In Reiki III you learn a new, fourth symbol called the master symbol. This is an expression of one's real self, the one with which you become one at the time of enlightenment. The symbol means, 'Great Being of the universe, please shine on me and be my friend,' and when used with Reiki it strengthens one's connection with one's higher self, resulting in manifestation on the material plane of the infinite power and wisdom of God. In addition to protecting the healing work being done, it brings Reiki energy together at one point and lends permanence to Reiki's positive results. The effects of the other three Reiki symbols are more pronounced when used in conjunction with this symbol, as it works at a much higher frequency than the others and taps into a much higher level of divine power; it brings a sense of completeness, fulfilment and wholeness. The master's symbol should be used *before* the other three symbols.

Chant the secret name of this symbol thrice, either verbally or mentally. Now repeat the following affirmation thrice:

'I establish my divine presence on this planet.'

Keep repeating each of the four symbols with this affirmation, and feel the power created in your being.

Benefits of Reiki III:

Meditation with Manifestation
Like all other meditation techniques, this powerful meditation exercise provides deep relaxation to your body, amazing clarity

to your thinking process, improved ability to visualize, enhanced healing potential, awakening to higher consciousness, intuitive foresight apart from blissful tranquility and calm to the whole of your being. It can also be used to solve your problems and for manifesting your goals.

The steps involved are:

1. Sit with your spine erect but not tense. You can sit cross-legged, sit in padmasana, vajrasana or sukhasna, or even sit in a straight-backed chair. If possible, sit facing east.
2. Place your hands one above the other, preferably the left above the right in your lap. Alternately, just place your hands on your knees or thighs if you find it more comfortable. Close your eyes and keep them closed throughout the meditation.
3. Take a deep and complete breath and imagine that you are inhaling pure white light that is reaching each nook and corner of your body. Exhale through your mouth, imagining that you are expelling all the rubbish released by this white light from all over the body. Take two more breaths in this way.
4. Draw the master symbol with the middle finger of your dominant hand, imagining violet light emanating out of it. Having drawn the symbol, hold it in your mental eye and repeat its name thrice. Hold the image of the symbol in your mind's eye for five to ten minutes. If your attention wavers, bring it back to the symbol as soon as you become aware of your distraction.
5. If you find it hard to hold the picture of the symbol in your mind's eye, hold the written symbol in your hand before you start the exercise, and open your eyes momentarily to look at it. Focus on that for a little while before closing your eyes again; this may help you retain the image.
6. After five to ten minutes, imagine the symbol moving from your field of vision into the field of white light above you.
7. Repeat steps 4 to 6 with the power symbol, mental/emotional healing symbol and distance healing symbol respectively.

8. At this point you may decide to finish the meditation and open your eyes. If you want to carry on for the purpose of manifesting your goals (which can be anything positive, from a change in job to more effective results for the healing you are providing someone), move on to step 9.

9. Make a mental picture of your goal having already been accomplished, and surround it with the four symbols. Imagine the master symbol on top, the power symbol on the right, the mental/emotional healing symbol on the bottom and the distant healing symbol on the left.

10. Hold this for five to ten minutes, then mentally say: 'If the fulfilment of this goal is permissible within your [Reiki's] divine love and wisdom, I pray that you let it be so.'

11. Imagine the image of your fulfilled goal (with the four symbols surrounding it) moving from your field of vision into the field of white light above you.

12. Feel the appropriate sense of accomplishment. Know with full, unshakable confidence that even though it may not manifest itself just yet, the goal has already been accomplished (just as an image is captured when you press the button on your camera, but what remains is only film that must be processed for the image to reveal itself).

13. If you wish, repeat steps 9 to 12 with any other goal(s) that you want manifested in the world of form.

14. If you find it difficult to make or hold mental pictures of your goals, do this exercise by writing your goal (or a picture of it) on a piece of paper and drawing the four symbols as described in step 9. Hold the paper in your hands and let the white light (emanating from your hands and your heart chakra) cover the paper.

15. To conclude the manifesting-goals-meditation, roll your tongue up to touch your palate and shift your attention to the back of the hara. Draw the power symbol on the front of your body, with the circular part on the front hara. Name the power symbol while patting your stomach thrice, in order to release any excess energy that might have been produced in your hara.

16. Open your eyes very slowly, to become only progressively aware of your surroundings.

THE HISTORY OF REIKI

Hindus believe that Lord Shiva blessed our planet with Reiki. Hence, Reiki can be seen as part of the common heritage of all humankind. We all tend to grab our toe in our hands if we stub it; a child does the same for her knee when she accidentally falls and scrapes it; a mother holds her baby on her lap and keeps her hands on his forehead when she finds him running a temperature. We tend to apply the warmth of our hands to any injured part of the body almost instinctively. Why do we do this if not as a response from our unconscious vestigial memory, from a time when the potential to heal through Reiki was part of the common human heritage?

It is believed that Reiki was brought to the Indian subcontinent by people from the Mu civilization. Though the Mu and Atlantis civilizations vanished with time, Reiki continued to be practised in India and Tibet. Gradually Reiki was lost here as well; only a handful of people passed it on from one generation to the next.

Reiki was practically lost altogether until it was rediscovered by Dr Mikaomi Usui, in Japan, towards the end of the nineteenth century.

Mikaomi Gyoho Usui (commonly known as Mikao Usui) was born on 15 August 1864 in a village called Yago, in the Yamagata district of Gifu in southern Japan. The son of Uzaemon, secretary to the mayor of Tokyo, Usui had a doctorate in literature, spoke many languages and had a deep interest in medicine, theology and philosophy. After marrying Sadako Suzuki, he had a son and a daughter. He once tried his hand at business, but he failed and was left in heavy debt. It was during these days of turmoil that Usui started looking for something with a deeper intrinsic meaning than material worth. Some believe this inclination towards spirituality was due not to his loss in business but to a spiritual awakening he had had during

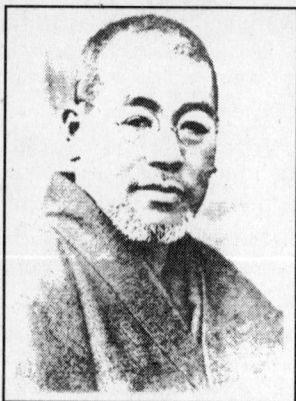

Mikao Usui

a near-death experience. After survating a bout with cholera around 1890, Usui got involved with a group named Rei Jyutsu Ka, based at the foot of Mt Kurama Yama, and meditated regularly next to a waterfall. Insatiably hungry for knowledge, he spent much of his time in Kyoto's libraries and monasteries studying ancient Buddhist medical texts. He experimented with every new technique he came across, and before long he was a well known Buddhist teacher with a large following. He often prayed to be guided towards a simple yet highly effective healing technique that could be learnt by one and all, irrespective of religious or educational background.

His prayers were granted: at the turn of the century, he accidentally discovered an ancient Buddhist manuscript (entitled *The Tantra of the Lightning Flash*) that revealed precisely such a technique. This system had been handed down from the time of Gautama Buddha, and practised in Tibet in the 7th century. Usui took his new-found treasure to Mt Kurama Yama to contemplate and understand it fully. His efforts were rewarded: during this retreat he received images and empowerments directly from the Reiki energy itself. He spent the next several years studying and refining his discoveries, and gathering them into a method that could be taught to the masses. This is how Rei-ki was re-born.

Having tried Reiki on his nearest and dearest, Usui was delighted with its efficacy and wanted to share it with others. For the next seven years he used Reiki to serve the downtrodden in and around Kyoto. In April 1921 he opened a clinic called Usui Reiki Ryoho Gakkei (Usui Reiki Healing Method Society) in Tokyo. The following year he founded a Reiki society, Usui Shiki Reiki Kenkyukai, which exists to this day. To make Reiki more effective, Usui incorporated five principles propagated by the emperor of Meiji, whom he held in high esteem; these principles are discussed in Chapter 5.

On 1 September 1923, the Kanto earthquake caused great devastation in Tokyo, leaving more than a lakh dead and tens of thousands injured. Dr Usui healed and brought relief to as many as he could through his clinic, but soon found that his present clinic could not handle all those seeking help. He opened another clinic at Nakano, outside Tokyo, and invitations started pouring in from all over Japan. His busy schedule over the next few years took its toll on his own health: while in Fukuyama on 9 March 1926, honouring an invitation, Usui had a heart attack (he had survived two such attacks earlier) and left for his heavenly abode. He is buried with his wife and son at Saihoji Buddhist temple on the outskirts of Tokyo.

Usui taught Reiki to almost two thousand students and trained between fourteen and nineteen teachers (records vary) in his lifetime. He often used crystals charged with Reiki to heal specific diseased areas. The focus of Usui's clinics was on healing, so the master symbol was rarely used. Distant healing was prevalent in Usui's time but was restricted to the rich, as only they could afford to have their photographs taken. The spread of Reiki after Usui's death was carried on by his senior disciples, such as Ogawa, Taketomi, Watanabe, Wanami, (the last three have been president of Usui's clinic in Tokyo) and Ms Koyama, who continues as the president of the clinic today. (It was Watanabe to whom Usui entrusted his personal notes, diaries and collection of Buddhist texts.) Recent research suggests that Usui's system of healing was quite a bit simpler than the one that we practise today.

The Western version of Dr Mikao Usui's story—better known than the above, but alas, dubious—holds that he was actually a Christian minister and the head of Doshisha University, in Kyoto. His students asked him constantly to show them the way to heal the body the way Jesus had healed others. Finally, Usui resigned from the university and embarked on a ten-year quest for the answer. Finding Japan's Christian authorities ignorant on this subject, he departed for the U.S., where he found the same problem. He enrolled at the University of Chicago Divinity School, studied comparative religions and philosophy and received a doctorate in theology. It was probably here that he learned to read Sanskrit.

Usui then travelled to India and Tibet before returning to Japan, where he moved into a Zen monastery near Kyoto. In the monastery's library Usui found an extensive collection of old Buddhist texts, and the abbot gave him unhindered access. Starting with Japanese texts and moving on to their Chinese counterparts, Usui continued his quest for precise healing formulas until he came to some old Buddhist texts in Sanskrit that finally seemed to hold what he was looking for. All he needed now was to learn how to activate the power within him to energize the symbols in the texts. This is what inspired him to spend twenty-one days on Mt Kurama Yama, which was about twenty-four kilometers from the monastery.

On reaching the mountain, Usui collected twenty-one small stones, placed them in front of him and threw away one at the end of each day. On the morning of the twenty-first day, while it was still dark, he saw a ball of strong light approaching him from a distance. So strong was the light that Usui thought of running away, lest it may strike and kill him, but he decided to trust it. Death or enlightenment—he was ready to receive either of the two, as enlightenment was his sole goal in life now. The light struck his third eye and knocked him down. When he regained consciousness a few moments later, he found himself surrounded by countless bubbles, all moving from right to left in all the seven colours of the rainbow. At the end came golden bubbles with white lights, and within the heart of each white light was a golden symbol in Sanskrit.

As Usui gathered himself and focused on each of the symbols, one by one, he received instructions on how to use the symbols he'd already discovered to activate the energy within him and to heal himself and others. He was still so afraid that he stopped blinking, lest he lose some important information. This is how the first Reiki master teacher was born, and how the lost ancient system of Reiki energy healing was reborn.

Usui ran down the mountain in his haste to tell the abbot he had finally been empowered. On the way, he stumbled and stubbed his toe. He instinctively sat down and held his toe in his hands, only to find it instantly healed. The bleeding stopped miraculously and the pain vanished. Near the foot of the mountain was a place where food was served to pilgrims, and alhough it is inadvisable to eat a full meal after such a long fast as Usui had undergone, he now had a full meal with no discomfort. Later, he also healed the girl serving the meals, who had endured a toothache for many days which had turned extremely severe that particular day. She was too poor to go to Kyoto to seek the help of a dentist. On reaching the monastery, he found the abbot in bed with arthritis; Usui placed one hand on the abbot's back and the other on his hips, and the abbot's pain simply vanished. Usui named this healing energy Reiki and meditated, along with the abbot, asking for guidance on the next course of action.

As a result of the guidance that dawned on them, Usui set out the next morning for the local leper colony. He stayed there for seven years, serving and healing most of the lepers in that time. After a few years, however, Usui began to see familiar faces—beggars he had healed years ago were returning. On inquiring, he found that they had come back to the leper colony because they were finding it difficult to earn their livelihood through discipline and hard work. Never before had they had to work for a living; they were not ready to start the new life Usui had meant for them. Now Usui realized his mistake: physical healing does not last if it is not backed by spiritual healing. Reiki given as charity to others only makes beggars of them. (By the word 'beggar', Usui meant anyone who wants to take without giving anything in return.) Usui decided that day that Reiki should never be given away without being given back in some form—the process of energy exchange. He left the leper colony, returned to Kyoto and decided to make the five principles of Reiki an integral part of the Reiki system of healing.

This Western version of Usui's story does not appear to be

true. No record at Doshisha University or the University of Chicago Divinity School shows that he was ever enrolled, and there is no evidence even to suggest he was a Christian. What might be true in this story is that Usui befriended some American Christian missionaries visiting Japan, who brought with them knowledge of Western medicine. It is likely that Usui was at one time invited to speak at the Christian school Doshi-Sha, in Kyoto, founded by a Japanese Christian in 1876. Usui's twenty-one-day retreat for meditation and fasting on Mt Kurama Yama may also be plausible, as this was indeed Usui's favourite place. Usui's diaries reveal that he received certain images (probably Reiki symbols) and Reiki empowerments directly through the Reiki energy itself, and the inscription on his tombstone makes a passing mention of his having attained a deep spiritual experience (*satori*) at Mt Kurama Yama. The experience said to have led Usui to introduce the concept of energy exchange might also be true, but the people he was serving in Kyoto between 1914 and 1921 were just downtrodden, not necessarily lepers.

The story of Reiki after Usui's transition is, however, simple enough and clear of controversy. Usui's son and daughter were not interested in committing their lives to Reiki, so Usui had to choose a successor from among his students. He entrusted the job of leading other teachers and spreading Reiki to two of his students, Toshihiro Eguchi and Dr Chujiro Hayashi, a Methodist

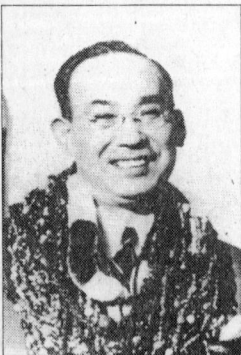

Chujiro Hayashi

Christian and commander in the imperial Japanese navy. After the transition, Hayashi opened a clinic in Tokyo and trained sixteen Reiki practitioners to treat all kinds of ailments therein. He modified the format of Usui's teachings and introduced the sytem of degrees and a different set of hand positions. As energy exchange, he would ask for three months, nine months and two years of unpaid assistance to initiate students progressively into the three degrees of Reiki. Like Usui, Hayashi had a son and daughter with other professional plans, so he chose Hawayo Takata as his successor before he left this world of form.

Hawayo Takata was born in 1900 on the island of Kauai, Hawaii. In 1917, working as a bookkeeper at a plantation owner's house, she met and married Saichi Takata, the plantation accountant. In 1930 she lost him, and the years following her husband's death were full of struggle. Her gall bladder needed surgery but she could not elect it, as she also suffered from respiratory problems that made anaesthesia inadvisable. Of Japanese origin, Takata went to Japan in 1935 to break the news of her sister's death to her parents, who had returned to Tokyo. Her own health was deteriorating, as she had now developed appendicitis and a tumour. She was admitted to Maeda Orthopaedic Hospital. The night before her surgery, she heard a voice saying the operation was not necessary. She heard the same voice again while lying on the operating table, just before the surgery started. Takata could not ignore the call any more—she asked Dr Maeda, the surgeon, whether the operation was really necessary. Maeda suggested she visit Hayashi's clinic, where her own sister had once learnt Reiki.

Six months later, Takata was completely healed. She now wanted to learn Reiki herself. Hayashi was reluctant to teach her, feeling that Reiki should be kept inside Japan, but he agreed to attune and train her for

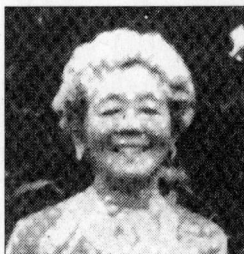

Hawayo Takata

Reiki I on the recommendation of Dr Maeda, who happened to be his uncle. After she had worked with the clinic's healers for a year, Takata received Reiki II and returned to Hawaii. In 1938, Hayashi came to Hawaii to confer Reiki III on her, and at that time he declared her his successor. Takata had to sell her home—her only possession with significant material value— to raise the $10,000 that Hayashi set as his fee for giving her a

Reiki mastership. This great exchange is an example of the commitment a Reiki master must make. She was now successfully running a clinic in Hawaii, and once she became a master she opened another one.

Two years later, in 1941, Takata saw an apparition—Hayashi was calling her back to him. On reaching Tokyo, Hayashi told her he was confronting a dilemma: he believed war would break out very soon, and as a reserve naval officer he would be called on to fight. As a healer, he was not supposed to take life. Hayashi resolved this dilemma by stopping his heart through psychic means and died on 10 May 1941, in the presence of his students. His body showed no signs of decay as it lay in state for a week at his Reiki clinic, and people from all over the country came to pay their respects.

Hayashi was proved right. The Second World War broke out, and with it, Reiki and its practitioners vanished from Japan. It was because Hayashi had foreseen this that he decided to make Takata—a foreigner—his successor. After the war, Takata was the sole thread through which Reiki continued and flourished: over the next four decades she trained hundreds of people and took Reiki to the United States, Canada and Europe. In the 1950s Takata became friends with the tobacco heiress Doris Duke and trained many of Duke's friends in Reiki, including the British writer Aldous Huxley. In the 1970s she started teaching extensively in the U.S., and in 1976 she made Virginia Samdahl, a healer and a teacher of metaphysics, her first Reiki master teacher. She trained twenty-two more Reiki masters by the time she died on 12 December 1980, naming Phyllis Lei Furumoto, her granddaughter, her successor along with a woman named Barbara Weber Ray. Takata taught each of these twenty-two masters differently, but she always insisted on charging a fee for Reiki, even from close relatives. She felt this was necessary to make people value Reiki.

After almost a year of working together, Barbara and Furumoto parted ways, and the Reiki movement split in two directions: the Reiki Alliance, led by Furumoto, and the Radiance Technique (also known as AIRA, or the American International

Reiki Association), led by Barbara Weber Ray. Both movements are still based in the U.S. In the early 1980s, Brigitte Muller brought Reiki to Europe, and in 1989 Dr Paula Horan, an American psychologist, brought Reiki to India. (Some, however, believe that Reiki was known and practised in the Rajneesh Ashram long before that.)

Methods now vary from teacher to teacher, and branches of Reiki have mushroomed. Some give Reiki III in two parts, III-A (the master practitioner) and III-B (the master teacher), while others give it as one consolidated credential. Some recommend spending a few months in Reiki I before moving on to Reiki II; others give both attunements on the same day.

Traditional Reiki masters call themselves purer because they believe that they are passing on Reiki in an unadulterated form. Non-traditional Reiki teachers proclaim that they are retaining the essentials of Reiki while refining, improving and adapting Reiki for modern times, based on their experience of what works best. I have nothing against enriching Reiki, but what makes a difference is how qualified the person trying to enrich Reiki is. By 'qualified' I mean whether he is himself a part of the pure lineage—the lineage that goes back to Mikao Usui without a break and whether he is himself a master in the real sense of the word. The one who is not a master, who is still to transcend his ego, is in danger of adding something to Reiki only whimsically, just to gratify his ego.

Some masters like to be addressed as 'grand masters' to distinguish themselves from the others. This only indicates that they are yet to overcome the petty but common human desire to seek gratification for our ego, instead of understanding and thus transcending this urge. Every particle of every river is where it is supposed to be at any point in time before it finally merges with the ocean; no particle is superior to the others. In fact, a Reiki grand master is responsible only for organization—keeping Reiki masters in touch with each other, arranging teachers' conferences—and for maintaining the purity and continuity of the school to which he belongs. No extra initiation, attunement, symbols or mantras are required to become a Reiki grand master;

the name only signifies experience and competence. In any case the term lost its technical relevance in 1988, as master attunement can now be passed on by any bona fide master teacher (one who has attained Reiki III or Reiki III-B, depending on the system in use). Until 1988, the master's attunement could only be given by a more senior master or a grand master, but now the same master who initiates one into Reiki I or II can initiate one into Reiki III as well.

3

Reiki Practice

Now that you have been introduced to Reiki, it is time to learn the basics of Reiki practice. Refer back to this part of the book whenever you have doubts or want to refresh your knowledge of certain techniques. At such moments, of course, especially during a healing session, your primary effort should be to bring more calm within your being so you are open and sensitive enough to any intuitive guidance that might be coming to you.

We begin by learning the sequence of hand positions that make up a full-body Reiki session, and the effects of each one. We shall then learn what constitutes a complete healing session, how to interpret the sensations that arise during Reiki, how group Reiki works, whether you should charge a fee when you treat others, how to combine Reiki with other healing methods, and how to integrate Reiki with your diet. We conclude with the principles of healing.

HAND POSITIONS

Reiki energy flows more smoothly and effectively within the healee's body when the practitioner follows a definite sequence of hand positions. There may be minor variations from teacher to teacher, but on the whole this sequence resembles the one followed by the flow of Reiki in the body.

I want to emphasize that merely placing the hands in the positions indicated does not bring about results *unless* you have been attuned by a bona fide Reiki master.

To administer any of these positions: hold both hands with palms down, facing the body of the patient. Extend and hold the fingers and thumb together, making an arch, so that a hollow is created under the palms as shown. Splayed fingers or flat palms might allow the energy to dissipate. Do not let the recipient cross his/her legs or arms.

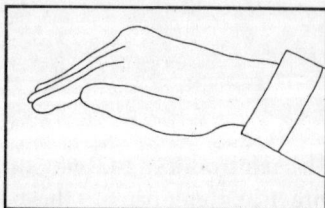

The hand positions below are the ones most Reiki masters teach and practise. I have made only a few modifications based on my own healing experience, particularly in emphasizing the feet. I identify three different hand positions for just one foot because I have found that, although most Reiki books mention only one, the reflex zones for almost the entire body are located at the feet. Whenever you don't have much time, or you don't want to touch the area you need to treat because it has been burnt or bruised, providing Reiki to these three positions is a great alternative. (You can also give Reiki to burnt or bruised locations by holding your palms an inch or so away from the body.) To break things up and make it easier to remember the positions, I divide the full-body treatment into four groups of seven positions each—head, torso, legs and back—as shown.

Group	Region	Details
A	Head	1. Eyes 2. Temples 3. Ears 4. Forehead 5. Occipital lobes 6. Throat 7. Thyroid
B	Torso	1. Heart 2. Solar plexus 3. Liver / Gall bladder 4. Lung tips 5. Pancreas/spleen 6. Naval/hara 7. Groin (spermatical cords or ovaries)
C	Legs	1. Knees 2. Right ankle 3. Right toes and toe ball 4. Right heel and arch 5. Left ankle 6. Left toes and toe ball 7. Left heel and arch
D	Back	1. Shoulders 2. Back of thyroid 3. Back of heart 4. Back of solar plexus 5. Kidneys / Adrenal glands 6. Back of hara 7. Root chakra

GROUP A: HEAD POSITIONS

Group A, the head positions, can best be covered while sitting or standing behind the patient's head. The patient can sit upright on a chair, or lie down on his or her back on a massage table or a mattress placed on the floor.

Position 1: Eyes

To treat yourself: Cup the eyes with your palms, with your fingers on the forehead and the sides of your palm comfortably placed on the sides of the nose. Let the smallest finger of each hand meet at the third eye.

To treat others: Sit or stand behind the head and place your arched palms on the eyes. The thumbs of both hands should touch near the middle of the eyebrows. Place your fingers comfortably on the sides of the patient's nose, taking care not to hinder or constrict the nostrils.

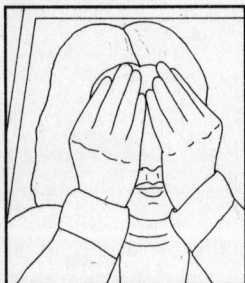

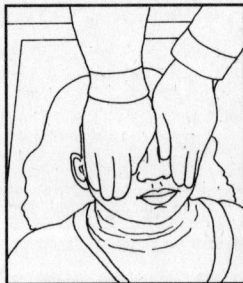

Chakra involved: Third eye.

Physical benefits: Relieves eye strain and arrests any weakening of the vision (if treatment is provided regularly for about 20 minutes at a time). May help heal any other eye problems such as glaucoma, cataracts, detached retina, etc., and problems relating to the pineal or pituitary glands. Sinuses, colds, flu, allergies and coughs can also improve. Sight, taste and smell get more sensitive.

Mental and emotional benefits: Growing awareness of one's real purpose in life, resulting in identification of one's real needs in all aspects of life. Feeling of peace and calm. Relief from discontent and possibly from addiction,

Spiritual benefits: Enhanced intuition and clairvoyance.

Position 2: Temples

To treat yourself: Place your palms on your temples (between your eyes and ears). The heel of each palm should be somewhere between the eye and the earlobe.

To treat others: Place your palms on the temples, with the tips of your fingers reaching the cheekbones. Keep your fingers and the thumbs together.

Alternately, let the fingers (in self-treatment) or the heels of the palms (in treating others) touch, but not overlap, on the top of the head.

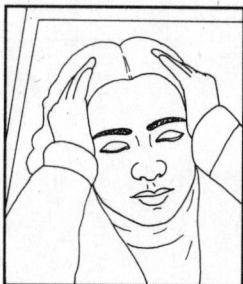

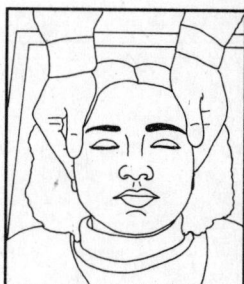

Chakra involved: Crown.

Physical benefits: Relaxes eye muscles, local nerves and other muscles radiating out from the jaw. May help heal colds, headaches, earaches and problems relating to the pineal or pituitary glands.

Mental and emotional benefits: Brings tranquillity by healing depression, manic depression or general anxiety. Strengthens the self from within—heals hate, dislike, anger, guilt or disgust towards oneself. Heals the inability to accept life as it unfolds (with all its fear, envy, sadness, disappointment, conflicts and other unpleasant happenings). Dissolves feelings of being unloved, disapproved of, rejected or anything else that blocks the self-esteem. Enables one to release pain or anger and forgive others. Helps maintain balance and coordination between the hemispheres of the brain, i.e., between logic and emotion. Improves creativity, memory, concentration and learning disabilities.

Spiritual benefits: Gradually wakes one up to the higher consciousness. May be used to assist someone dying.

Position 3: Ears

To treat yourself: Place your cupped palms on your ears.

To treat others: Same as above.

Alternately, hold this position but move the index fingers into the ear holes.

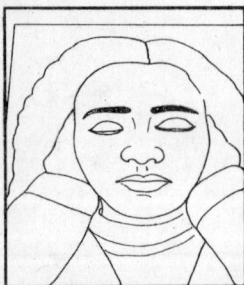

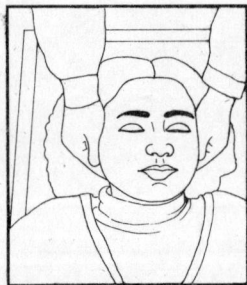

Chakra involved: Third eye.

Physical benefits: The ears are an important Reiki position for any kind of ailment, as the ears keep our bodies in balance. Like the palms of the hands and the soles of the feet, the ears are 'circuit boards' comprising nerve endings from most major parts of the body; they hold a number of important acupuncture points connecting all the major energy meridians. Providing

Reiki at this position can improve hearing loss, balance problems and—because the ears are connected to the nasal and pharyngeal regions—colds. The receiver feels immediate relaxation.

Mental and emotional benefits: Helps develop intuition and the ability to resolve conflicts. Improves self-esteem by healing the feeling of being unloved, deserted, abandoned or devoid of emotional support. Develops the ability to deal with anger in a positive way by accepting life as it unfolds. Dissolves the resistance to listen to and consider others' views and opinions.

Spiritual benefits: Brings mind, body and spirit into balance.

Position 4: Forehead

To treat yourself: Place one hand on your forehead and the other at the back of the head, opposite the first. Keep your fingers and thumbs together.

To treat others: Same as above.

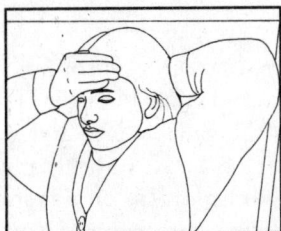

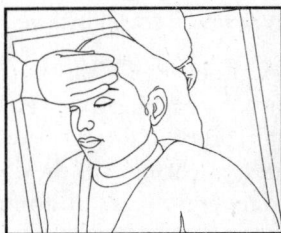

Chakra involved: Third eye.

Physical benefits: Relieves headaches and related tensions.

Mental and emotional benefits: Heals anger, disappointment, anxiety and frustration. Enables one to evaluate oneself without fear and learn from one's experiences. Helps improve intuition. Redirects intellectual skills towards positive pursuits.

Spiritual benefits: Improves understanding of spiritual matters.

Position 5: Occipital Lobes

The occipital lobe is the rearmost lobe in each hemisphere of the brain.

To treat yourself: Cup the occipital lobes where the throat meets the lower back of the skull.

To treat others: Cradle the back of the head in your relaxed palms. The sides of the palms should touch, with the fingers reaching the base of the skull.

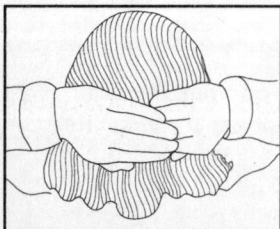

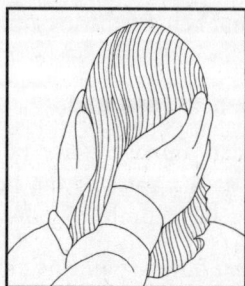

Chakra involved: Third eye.

Physical benefits: Heals headaches, circulatory disorders and problems stemming from cerebellum and spinal fluid, the brain's visual cortex, the large intestine, the gall bladder and what Chinese medicine calls the governor vessel. Helps heal asthma, headaches, colds, abdominal complaints, emphysema, pneumonia, hyperventilation, sneezing, nausea and insomnia and other sleep disorders.

Mental and emotional benefits: Calms the mind. Helps develop balance and coordination between the hemispheres of the brain (i.e., between logic and emotion) and between the pituitary and pineal glands. Heals the old reptilian brain that regulates involuntary support functions such as breathing, heartbeat, muscle movement and digestion. May facilitate past-life recall and dream recall.

Spiritual benefits: Heals addictive behavioural patterns and third-eye blockages. Heals absent-mindedness.

Position 6: Throat

To treat yourself: Slide one hand under the hollow of the neck and bring the other over the front of the throat. Keep the fingers and thumbs of both hands together.

To treat others: Same as above. Let the edge of the upper palm take support from the patient's collarbone so he or she does not feel pressure on the wind pipe.

Alternately, the palms can be kept at sides of the throat.

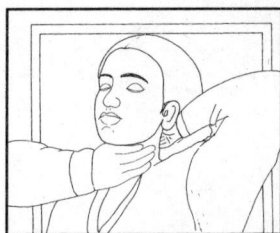

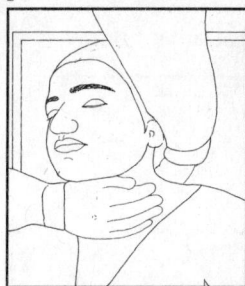

Chakra involved: Throat.

Physical benefits: Heals the vocal cords and specific speech problems such as hoarseness and stammering. Heals clogged sinuses, blood-pressure problems, metabolic diseases, weight problems, swollen glands, gum disease, throat and mouth ulcers, anorexia, osteoporosis, palpitation, poor posture, shoulder tension, problems in the pelvic region and legs, sore throat, laryngitis, tonsilitis and other throat ailments, and problems relating to the thyroid and parathyroid glands (for the assimilation of calcium and magnesium).

Mental and emotional benefits: Heals under- or over-expression of aggression and the inability to express one's true feelings, thoughts or beliefs. Builds confidence and enhances self-esteem and creativity; heals stage fright. Makes one communicate better, work more systematically and bring order into one's life.

Spiritual benefits: Helps one know one's purpose in life and direct one's energies towards fulfilling one's dreams. Heals addictive behavioural patterns and third-eye blockages.

Position 7: Thyroid

To treat yourself: Place one palm over the small depression at the bottom of the throat and the other just adjacent to and below it. In these positions, the upper and lower hands cover the thyroid and thymus glands respectively.

To treat others: Same as above.

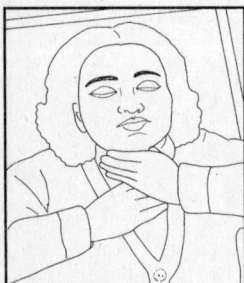

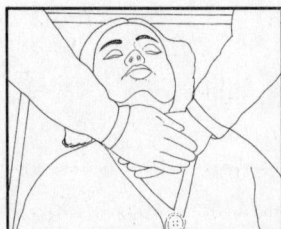

Chakra involved: Throat.

Physical benefits: Improves circulation and immunity.

Mental and emotional benefits: Enables one to speak and live by one's own truth, to give and take graciously and to bring clarity and order to one's life.

Spiritual benefits: Improves sensitivity to one's inner voice. Helps one stand up to one's responsibilities and fulfill one's needs.

GROUP B: TORSO POSITIONS

If you are giving Reiki to someone else, these positions will be easier if you stand on one side of the torso.

Position 8: Heart

To treat yourself: Continuing from Position 7, keep your lower hand where it is but move the upper one below it, still adjacent.

To treat others: Same as above. However, when treating a woman, place one hand between the breasts and the other horizontally just above it (over the thymus gland), forming a T. If you are a male and not on intimate terms with your patient, keep your hands an inch or so above the breasts as a mark of respect for a woman's privacy. You can also use this T variation for males if your intuition guides you to do so, or if you simply find yourself more comfortable with it.

Alternately, place your left palm over your right palm above the heart. Though it is the heart chakra (placed right in the centre) and not the physical heart (which is slightly towards one's left), allow your hands to be guided a bit to one side by any pull or repulsion they experience.

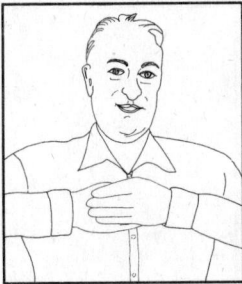

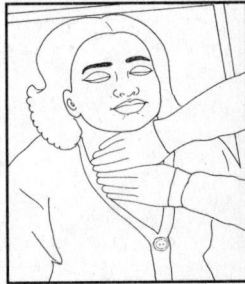

Chakra involved: Heart.

Physical benefits: Helps heal cardiac problems, asthma, pneumonia, deafness, lung cancer and auto-immune disorders such as arthritis, chronic fatigue, general weakness, AIDS, cancer and so forth. Strengthens immune system and improves circulation and respiratory health.

Mental and emotional benefits: Removes resistance to receiving or giving love. Heals excessive need for approval by others. Enhances feelings of trust and harmony. Heals emotional problems—grief, guilt, feelings of betrayal, inability to forgive, depression, and so forth. Heals lack of emotion and excess emotion.

Spiritual benefits: Wakes one up to God's subtle love, manifested all around us. Awakens lost compassion and love. Starts one on the journey back to oneself.

Position 9: Solar Plexus

To treat yourself: Continuing from Position 8, keep your lower hand where it is and move the upper one below it, still adjacent.

To treat others: Same as above.
　Alternately, place the hands in a horizontal line across the solar plexus, across the depression where the lower ribs meet in front.

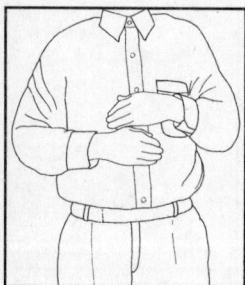

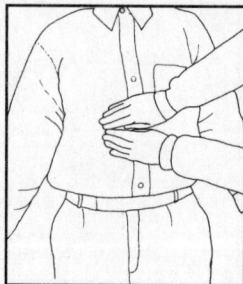

Chakra involved: Solar plexus.

Physical benefits: Heals the digestive organs (liver, stomach, gall bladder, spleen, alimentary canal) and thus helps heal digestive problems: gastric or duodenal ulcers, anorexia nervosa, bulimia, diabetes, colon and intestinal problems, arthritis, liver disorders, fat around the middle of the body.

Mental and emotional benefits: Heals the inability to trust others, the inability to take responsibility and make decisions, and power-struggle issues. Banishes fears. Helps heal nervous tension and problems with self-esteem, confidence, self-respect and self-control. Heals relationship issues and harmonises emotional and physical love.

Spiritual benefits: Develops intuition. Helps one discern one's connection to the grand plan of the universe.

Position 10: Liver / Gall Bladder

To treat yourself: Place your left hand just below your right-hand bottom-most rib, reaching up towards the middle of the body, and the other just adjacent and below it.

To treat others: Same as above.

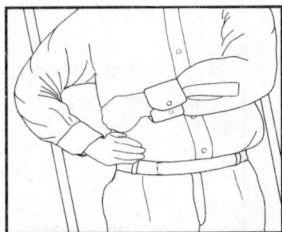

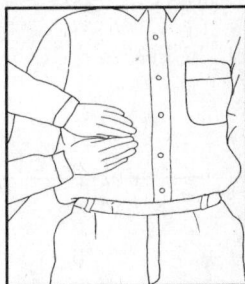

Chakra involved: Solar plexus.

Physical benefits: Releases toxins from the body. Heals liver problems (such as jaundice), gall-bladder problems, high blood pressure, hormonal imbalances, cholestrol problems, allergies, haemorrhoids, headaches and metabolic diseases.

Mental and emotional benefits: Heals spleen, anger and other repressed aggressive emotions. Improves decision-making ability.

Spiritual benefits: Improves relationships, especially with the masculine aspects of the universe (in the physical world, fathers and men generally). Accelerates spiritual growth, improves judgement and brings a harmonious balance to the way one lives. Fine-tunes the realtionship between ideals and what one actually practises.

Position 11: Lung Tips

To treat yourself: Place your fingertips on either side of your collarbone.

To treat others: Same as above, except that if you sit behind the patient's head rather than at his side, you will touch the collarbones with the heels of your palms rather than with your fingertips.

Alternately, place the hands in a horizontal line across the thymus. In treating yourself, the fingers should touch each other at the tips; in treating others, the fingers of one hand should touch the heel of the other palm.

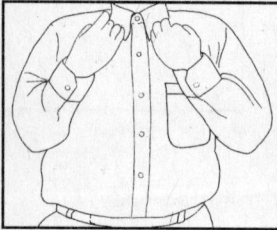

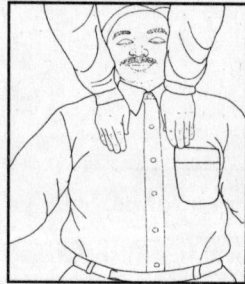

Chakra involved: Heart/Thymus.

Physical benefits: Helps heal lung problems. Particularly beneficial for smokers, people with asthma and people living in polluted cities.

Mental and emotional benefits: Fine-tunes emotional needs / expectations of love and the satisfaction received from relationships.

Spiritual benefits: Dissolves doubts about one's divinity (and resourcefulness) and thereby helps a sense of trust, space and freedom in one's life to flower.

Position 12: Pancreas/Spleen

To treat yourself: Place your right hand just below the left-hand bottom-most rib and the left hand adjacent to and below it. Same as Position 10 but on the left side.

To treat others: Same as above.

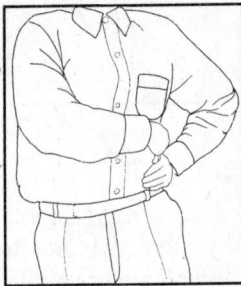

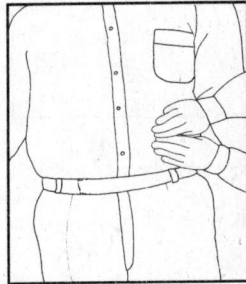

Chakra involved: Solar plexus.

Physical benefits: Helps heal indigestion, diabetes, hypoglycaemia, rheumatoid arthritis and all kinds of infections. Peps up one's energy level.

Mental and emotional benefits: Heals fears, suppressed anger, tendency to manipulate and/or be manipulated, and an excess or dearth of sweetness. Enhances self-esteem, helps one feel centered, and facilitates confident decision-making,

Spiritual benefits: Develops equanimity, tranquillity and trust in the beauty, sweetness, meaningfulness and perfection of life and the universe.

Position 13: Navel/Hara

To treat yourself: Place one hand above the navel and the other below it.

To treat others: Same as above.

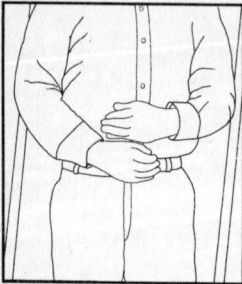

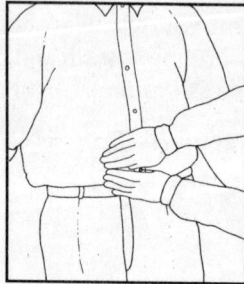

Chakra involved: Hara.

Physical benefits: Improves digestion. Helps heal metabolic and gastrointestinal diseases, nausea, bloating, haemorrhoids, prostate and bladder disorders, sexual and reproductive problems, cervical and prostate cancer, fibroids, tumours, allergies, pelvic and lower-back pain, skin disorders, addictions and overindulgence in alcohol, sex or food. Enhances vitality.

Mental and emotional benefits: Heals emotional scars, depression and anxiety. Improves intuition. Brings inner peace and harmony. May help bring suppressed feelings to the surface. (Men, because they tend to have more suppressed feelings than women, tend to draw more Reiki in this position.) Improves the ability to enjoy physical and sexual pleasures. Heals relationship problems and helps remove people, places, material things, situations and whatever is no longer required in your life. Drawing Reiki in this position, along with those for the root chakra, can help you switch to a career you love, one that is in true harmony with your purpose in life.

Spiritual benefits: Brings peace and stability. Awakens dormant creativity.

Position 14: Groin

To treat yourself: Form a V with your palms over the pelvic bones, and adjust until your hands cover the genitals. Keep your fingers and thumbs together.

To treat others: Same as above, but it might be more convenient to point the far hand in the opposite direction (i.e., point the closer hand towards the thighs and the farther hand away from them). Preserve your patient's privacy by keeping your hands just above his or her body.

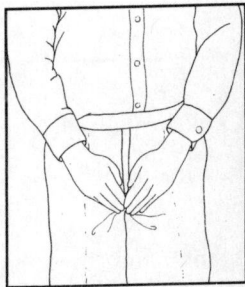

Chakra involved: Root.

Physical benefits: Heals physical and emotional problems relating to the urinary and reproductive systems. Improves appetite, immunity, circulation and digestion. May prevent the development of ovarian cysts and breast tumours in women and prostate problems in men. Also heals allergies, weight problems, migraine headaches, menopause problems and general weakness. Aids in convalescence.

Mental and emotional benefits: Resolves sexual issues, including fear of physical intimacy. Heals lack of will to live or to enjoy life.

Spiritual benefits: Makes one feel grounded and centered.

GROUP C: LEG POSITIONS

Position 15: Knees

To treat yourself: Assume a sitting posture and cup your knees with your hands.

To treat others: Same as above.

Alternately, treat each knee separately by placing both hands on one knee at a time— one above and the other at the back, in

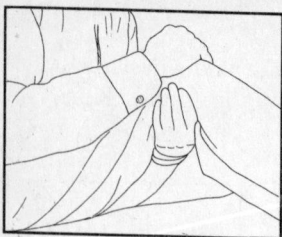

the hollow of the joint. This variation is preferable for those with stiff or weak knee joints, those under stress, those confronting and fearing a particular change in life or those who generally find it emotionally difficult to face life's challenges with courage.

Chakra involved: Minor chakras in the knee region.

Physical benefits: Helps heal arthritic knees and other knee problems.

Mental and emotional benefits: Helps dissolve stubbornness, arrogance, fear of death or any unyielding attitude that keeps us from letting go, moving ahead and facing change.

Spiritual benefits: Dissolves excessive fears and attachments relating to insecurity, uncertainty and prospects for change. Enhances humility, empathy, tolerance and forgiveness.

Position 16: Right Ankle

To treat yourself: Encircle your right ankle with your palms. The fingertips of one hand should touch the heel of the other palm.

To treat others: Same as above, but (for the sake of convenience) the fingertips of one hand should touch those of the other.

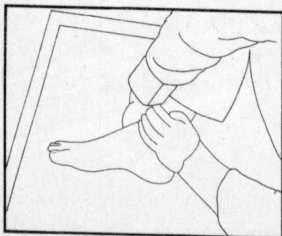

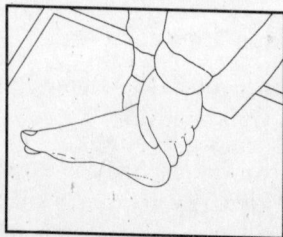

Chakra involved: Root.

Physical benefits: Helps heal problems in the digestive system, the pelvic joint and muscles, the ovaries or testes and the lymphatic system. Dissolves blocks in the flow of energy from the feet to the root chakra.

Mental and emotional benefits: Helps one learn to experience pleasure in life, to rejoice and be cheerful.

Spiritual benefits: Brings balance into one's life through a flexible attitude and a realization that it is futile to carry guilt around.

Position 17: Right Toes and Toe Ball

To treat yourself: Place your left palm along your right foot, under the toe ball and the toes. Then cover all the toes by lying your right palm across them.

To treat others: Same as above.

Chakra involved: Root.

Physical benefits: Strengthens the root chakra and helps heal colds, headaches and digestive problems. Can help relieve those recovering from coma, anaesthesia or any kind of shock.

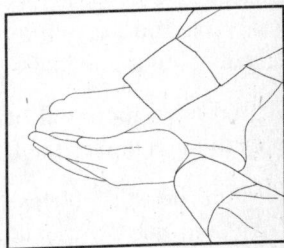

Since this position carries the reflex zones for the eyes, ears, shoulders, heart, thyroid and parathyroid glands, frontal sinuses, pituitary gland and neck, it can also heal problems relating to all these areas.

Mental and emotional benefits: Grounds all the chakras—that is, stabilizes their spin by connecting them to the centre of Mother Earth through a thin, laser-like column of energy.

Spiritual benefits: Connects one to the earth element.

Position 18: Right Heel and Arch

To treat yourself: Cup the back of your right ankle with your right palm. Place your left palm next to it, beneath the arch of the foot. Leave no gaps between the fingers, including the thumb.

To treat others: Same as above.

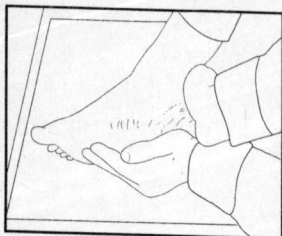

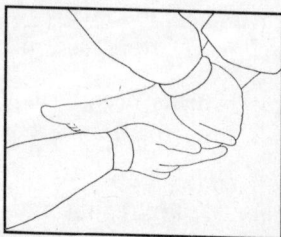

Chakra involved: Secondary foot chakra at the arch.

Physical benefits: This area covers reflex zones for the gonads, solar plexus, sciatic nerves, gall bladder, ureter, small intestine, transverse and ascending colon, duodenum, pancreas, kidneys, stomach, lungs and knees.

Mental and emotional benefits: Dissolves energy blocks and fears of moving into the future.

Spiritual benefits: Helps preserve one's connection with the earth, and thereby the ability to manifest one's dreams in the physical world.

Positions 19-21: Left Foot

Repeat positions 16-18 on the left foot.

The left foot covers reflex zones for the descending colon, spleen and liver, and thus provides healing energy to all of these organs.

GROUP D: BACK POSITIONS

The back represents support, both financial (lower back) and
emotional (upper back).

Position 22: Shoulders

To treat yourself: Place your palms over your shoulders, at the
sides of your neck. If you find this difficult, you may cross your
arms so that each palm touches the opposite shoulder.

Alternately, hold one palm over the opposite shoulder, near
the neck, and place the other palm over the kidney on that side.
Repeat on the other shoulder. If you adopt this variation, you
may skip the kidney position later on (Position 25).

To treat others: Place your palms over the shoulders, parallel
to each other. Alternately, place your palms in a straight
horizontal line across the shoulder blades, with the fingertips
of the hand closer to you touching the heel of the other palm.

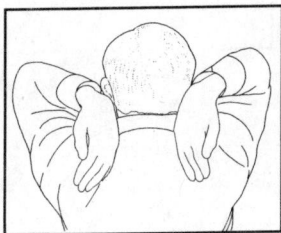

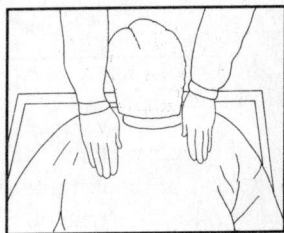

Chakra involved: Back of throat.

Physical benefits: Releases accumulated tension in the neck and
shoulder regions. Heals headaches and lung problems. Activates
the parasympathetic nervous system (which calms the body
when necessary) and, when combined with abdominal positions,
improves digestion through the autonomic nervous system.

Mental and emotional benefits: Releases stress and heals
responsibility issues, such as overestimating or failing to admit

one's personal responsibilities. Helps one initiate relationships that one has avoided for fear of rejection.

Spiritual benefits: Helps one develop the courage to discover one's purpose in life and apply oneself to it.

Position 23: Back of Thyroid

To treat yourself: Bring your palms together at the back of your neck, one on top of the other.

To treat others: Have the patient lie on his or her stomach, head towards you. Place your palms together, one on top of the other, on the little protrusion at the base of the neck.

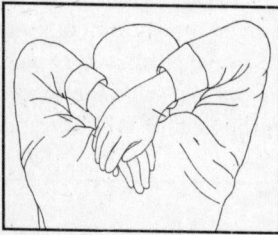

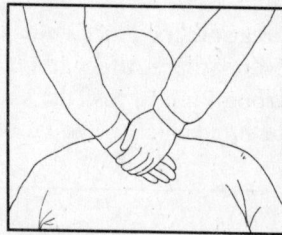

Chakra involved: Back of thyroid.

Physical benefits: Helps heal thyroid problems, neck stiffness, headaches, auto-immune diseases (not AIDS) and dental problems. Relieves general stress.

Mental and emotional benefits: As it relates to professional satisfaction, this position helps one discover one's calling or purpose in life, develop self-esteem and overcome fears of failure or rejection.

Spiritual benefits: Wakes one up to one's life purpose and unleashes a commitment to pursue it. Instead of looking for excuses and playing the role of a victim, one starts to take responsibility for one's circumstances. The objective shifts from surviving to thriving.

Position 24: Back of Heart

To treat yourself: Bring your palms back from their respective sides and thrust them up towards the heart level as far they can go. Upturn them, letting the backs of the palms touch the body.

Alternately, bring one hand from the top over the corresponding shoulder and the other up from below, to meet behind the heart. Both palms should face the body.

These are not comfortable or convenient positions and cannot be assumed for long intervals. Reiki II provides further options for healing this chakra.

To treat others: Place your palms in a straight horizontal line across the shoulder blades, with the fingertips of one hand touching the heel of the other palm. The hands should be one

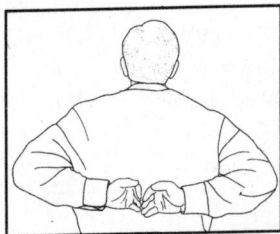

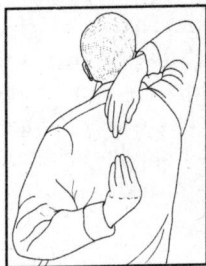

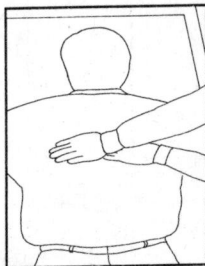

palm width below the alternative for Position 22. This back position corresponds to Position 8 in front.

Chakra involved: Back of heart.

Physical benefits: Helps heal heart and lung problems,

Mental and emotional benefits: Softens the heart emotionally. May heal manic depression.

Spiritual benefits: Wakes one up to the universal love, and to one's own love for the One who is the source of all love.

Position 25: Back of Solar Plexus

To treat yourself: Place both palms on your back at the level of the solar plexus, with fingertips touching. This position is difficult to hold for long, but Reiki II provides further options.

To treat others: Same as Position 23 but at the level of Position 9 in back. That is, place one arched hand on top of the other over the spine, at the level of the bottom-most ribs in front.

Alternately, same as Position 9 but at the back. Place your hands in a horizontal line across the spine, with the fingers of the closer hand touching the heel of the other at the level of the bottom-most ribs in front.

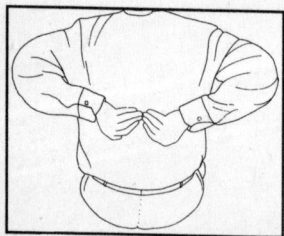

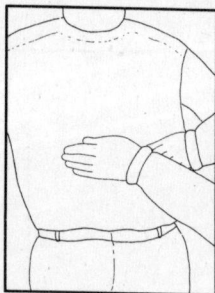

Chakra involved: Back of solar plexus.

Physical benefits: Heals colic and intestinal cramps, gastritis and middle-back pain.

Mental and emotional benefits: Helps heal issues with power, wisdom or control. Makes one realize one's responsibility to stay physically healthy, and awakens one to the emotional trash one is trying to hide from oneself.

Spiritual benefits: Bestows powers for spiritual healing.

Position 26: Kidneys / Adrenal Glands

To treat yourself: Place your palms in a horizontal line across your back, one palm width above the waist (in line with the lower ribs), fingertips touching.

To treat others: Same as above, but you may find it more convenient to point the fingertips of the far hand away from you (touch the fingertips of one hand to the heel of the other palm).

Chakra involved: Back of solar plexus / root.

Physical benefits: Heals kidney problems and helps prevent kidney failure in case of serious shock. Releases toxins. Can help heal fear of intimacy, sexual problems, infertility, allergies, acrophobia and reluctance to share one's feelings. Regular healing prolongs life and preserves youthfulness. Maintains digestive organs and sympathetic nerve balance.

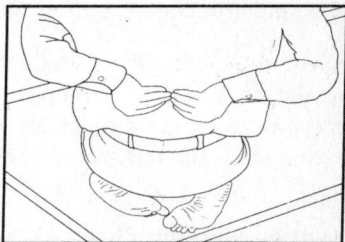

Mental and emotional benefits: Filters out ideas and concepts that have outgrown their utility. Relieves stress. Helps heal partnership or relationship problems.

Spiritual benefits: Heals relationships at a spiritual level. Empowers one by aligning one's personal will with God's will.

Position 27: Back of Hara

To treat yourself: Same as Position 26 but one palm width below,

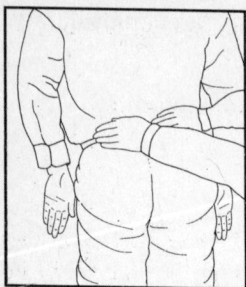

just above the buttocks.

To treat others: Same as above, but touch the fingertips of one hand to the heel of the other palm.

Chakra involved: Back of hara.

Physical benefits: Helps heal lower-back pain, problems with immunity, sexual problems, sciatic-nerve problems, and the backs of the small and large intestines.

Mental and emotional benefits: Heals fear of abandonment, emotional insecurity, low sex drive, fear of intimacy, aversion to sexual intercourse, sexual perversion and sexual addiction.

Spiritual benefits: Brings balance to one's relationships (with people, food, money, animals, the surroundings, Nature, the universe and oneself). Helps one see the meaning in each relationship and feel secure in it.

Position 28: Root Chakra

To treat yourself: Place both hands on the tailbone, with the right one touching the tailbone and the left one above it.

Alternately, bring your right hand from the front beneath the coccyx (the bottom-most triangular bone at the base of the spinal column) and the left hand from the back to cover the

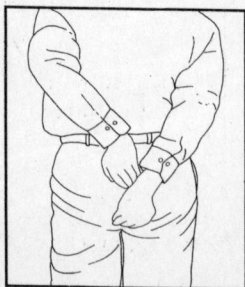

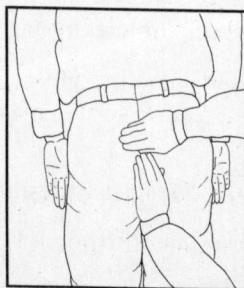

perineum (the area between the anus and the genitals).

To treat others: Place one hand over and along the fold of the buttocks and the other perpendicular to it, forming a 'T'.

Chakra involved: Root.

Physical benefits: Heals urogenital and digestive problems, chronic lower-back pain, sciatica and varicose veins. Can help treat fissures, rectal tumours and cancers.

Mental and emotional benefits: Strengthens the will to live. Helps one find effective ways to fulfil financial and other neeeds. Banishes fear; lends a sense of security and safety. Strengthens sense of commitment. Develops assertiveness. Heals long-time grudges towards parents.

Spiritual benefits: Connects one to Mother Earth and her abundance. One feels grounded and centered.

FULL-BODY REIKI

Going through all the above hand positions, on either yourself or your patient, constitutes full-body Reiki.

I once heard someone say that when your wife complains she has a headache, you should not hand her an aspirin; she just needs your attention, or a loving touch showing that you care. With Reiki you cannot make the 'aspirin' mistake, as you heal only through a loving touch. Most people will never be touched so elaborately in a lifetime as they could be in a full-body Reiki session. Those who give themselves regular full-body Reiki, without distraction, become sensitive to their own bodies and come to notice changes in the sensations their hands experience as they move from one part of the body to the next. You learn which parts of the body have blocks and which ones are open to receiving Reiki. (Writing your observations can further assist you in developing this consciousness.) Similarly, when you give Reiki to others you become even more distinctly aware of your own body's sensations. Full-body Reiki also helps anyone who is convalescing after serious illness or surgery, and it alleviates the harmful side effects of allopathic treatments such as chemotherapy (see 'Combining Reiki with Other Healing Methods', below, and the Reiki positions for cancer in Chapter 4).

Because each organ in the body is interconnected with the rest, our organs are interdependent. A weak pancreas can affect the energy configuration and pulsations of the left kidney, and affect the kidney's health unless something is done to restore the balance. Untreated indigestion can result in the accumulation of waste in the muscle tissues, the blood vessels and especially the joints, which in turn strains the kidneys and other organs of elimination and results in fatigue. The pillars of our invisible anatomy, i.e., the chakras, also affect each other—a malfunction in one chakra can put excessive strain on the others. If the chakras are out of sync, any existing aural imbalance can be aggravated. Under such circumstances, providing Reiki in just one or two places may have limited effects. Full-body Reiki (which usually takes about 90 minutes), along with chakra balancing and scanning, harmonizes the ailing being at all levels.

Thus, unless you labour under severe time constraints, you should treat every ailment with full-body Reiki before you focus on specific positions.

SCANNING

Scanning does to the whole aura what chakra balancing does to the chakras. As a Reiki channel you already have open palm chakras, and thus enhanced sensitivity to aural energy and its vibrations; in scanning, one hand is moved along the spine in search of any sudden change or distortion in the vibrations. If such a change is detected, it can be healed by holding both hands there and providing Reiki until the flow of Reiki subsides. Scanning should precede a healing session, as it facilitates the flow and absorption of Reiki during treatment.

The steps involved in scanning are:

1. Have the patient lie down on his back. Pray for guidance on

where he or she needs Reiki the most.

2. Hold your left (or non-dominant) hand about a foot above the patient's head. Note the sensations in your hand.

3. Slowly bring your hand down until it is about three inches above the head. Maintaining the same distance from the body, start gliding your hand very slowly along the spine (though still on the front of the body) until you reach the feet. Be aware of any fluctuations in the energy level or sensations in your palm—these indicate a need to hold your hand still and provide Reiki. Your palm may experience a pull, pressure (due to repulsion), coolness, warmth, tingling, pulsations or a feeble electric charge. When you feel the need to provide Reiki, stop your palm and move it slowly up and down in that location to find the point of maximum distortion. You may discover it as far as two feet from the body itself, though it's usually closer.

4. Let your right hand join your left hand to provide Reiki where necessary. Continue until you feel the flow of Reiki subside.

5. Resume gliding your left palm until you find another such spot. Stop at each such point to provide Reiki until you reach the feet.

6. Be constantly open to any intuitive guidance that might throw light on the causes of the energy distortion or suggest how the patient can address the problem at its root. Any such information should be disclosed to the patient with humility, and for the sole reason of your love for him or her, and with the utmost respect.

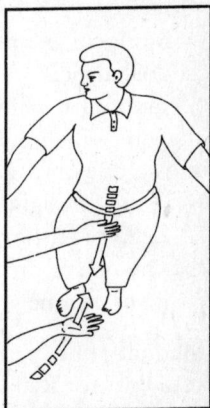

Self-Scanning: You can scan your own body, too. Self-scanning improves self-knowledge.. Revelations of what needs healing should be followed up with sincere soul-searching, but with a forgiving attitude rather than pangs of guilt.

BALANCING THE CHAKRAS

The pranic body receives energy from the environment and passes it on to the physical body through the chakras, via the endocrine system (the system of glands that maintain the body's hormonal balance). Each chakra corresponds to one gland located near it on the physical plane, and through that gland caters to the health of a group of corresponding organs. The endocrine glands and chakras are interdependent, so balancing the chakras through Reiki energy brings about hormonal balance as well.

When the energy flow through any of the chakras is too low or too high, perhaps due to a setback, stress or sudden, ecstatic joy, one's physical, mental and spiritual health can be adversely affected.

By opening up the chakras gradually and harmoniously, chakra balancing dissolves energy blocks and frees your dormant talents and capabilities. If regularly done first thing in the morning—before you even get up—chakra balancing will not only give you a good start, but will keep you centred and energetic throughout the day.

Reiki practitioners employ various methods to balance the chakras. Here are some of the most common; try them and settle on the one your intuition guides you to.

Method 1: Let your patient stand with his or her side towards you. Pray for Reiki to flow through your hands (unless you are already in the middle of a Reiki session). Place one hand a few inches in front of the root chakra, the other at its back. Pay attention to the sensations in your hands — what exactly are you feeling? Keep your hands still for a few minutes; you may feel the pulsations of a magnetic energy. Now move your hands up to the hara, and hold your hands on either end of this bipolar chakra; hold this position for a few minutes. Repeat with each chakra until you come to the monopolar crown chakra. Now hold your hands a few inches above your head, one above the other, taking care not to hold them directly above the fontanelle. Hold this position for about five minutes and then move back downwards until you reach the root chakra once more. If you are guided while your hands are on a particular chakra to hold that position longer, follow your intuition.

Method 2: Let the patient lie down on his or her stomach, and pray for Reiki to flow through your hands. Place one hand over the upper part of the head, right at the back of the third eye, and the other under the tailbone. Wait until you feel sensations in both hands, then close your eyes and focus on these sensations and their

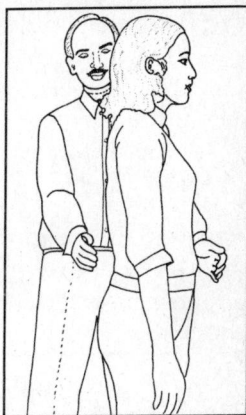

Method 1

intensity—warmth, tingling, pulsations, whatever. Now shift the hand that was under the tailbone to a position over the hara and the other to a position over the throat chakra. Feel the sensations, and wait for them to even up in both hands. Shift your hands to the solar-plexus and heart chakras to complete the process. Before you complete the process by slowly removing your hands from the solar-plexus and heart chakras, you might be intuitively guided to try various other combinations of chakras. If you are an advanced practitioner, you may want to use symbols as well.

Alternately, those who normally expend a lot of mental energy can place one hand on the third eye and move the other upwards, starting from the root chakra, always changing the position when both hands feel the same intensity of energy. If you find it hard to focus, and thus to feel sensations in your hands, try rubbing them before the treatment.

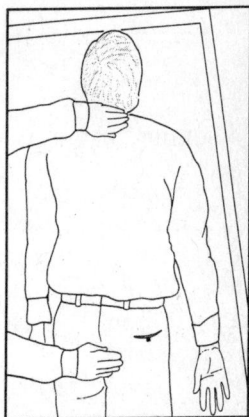

Method 2

To distribute the energy released during chakra balancing, follow this treatment with a smoothing of the aura (see below). Some practitioners balance the chakras after a Reiki session, but in the case of a sensitive patient, perform these two treatments *before* a Reiki session to help the patient relax completely and feel more open to the energy transfer ahead.

Method 3: If you are working with another Reiki channel, the two of you can try balancing the patient's chakras simultaneously. Place your hands on the first and sixth chakras and have your colleague place his or her hands on the second and fifth chakras. You may have to sit on opposite sides of the patient, who should lie on his or her back. The patient should place the left hand on the heart chakra and the right hand on the solar plexus. The patient does not have to be a Reiki channel, but you may have to smooth out the aura before and after the session in any case. Stroke the patient's energy by giving a loving touch all over the body. Ask the patient to lie still for a while after the treatment and come back to the waking state slowly.

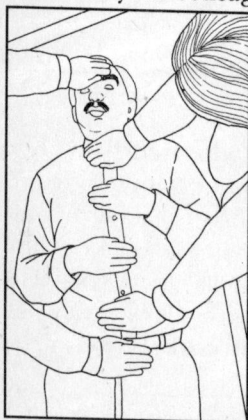

Method 3

SMOOTHING THE AURA

Smoothing the aura evens out any energy imbalances and ensures the harmonious flow of energy through the aura. It also helps prepare the healee by establishing amiable contact with his or her subconscious, akin to shaking hands before starting a conversation. This eases any feelings of intimidation and aids in receptivity.

To smooth a patient's aura:

1. Have the patient lie down supine.

2. Keeping your left hand on your own hara, make a quick sweep over your patient's body from head to toe with your right hand (palm facing patient's body), at a distance of half a foot. This communicates your being centered, as the left hand is the receiving hand while the right hand is the giving hand.

3. Keeping the palm vertical and close to the patient's body, move your right hand back to the head from the toes. This coveys your presence everywhere within him or her.

4. Repeat steps 2 and 3 two more times.

Follow the same procedure after the Reiki session is over, only this time keep your left hand on the patient's hara instead of your own. This conveys to the healee metaphysically that the session is over.

THE HEALING SESSION, COMPLETE AND WHOLE

A typical healing session proceeds as follows. This list is only for your guidance; feel free to skip or modify one or two steps if your intuition or experience guides you to do so.

(i) **Prepare the room:** Before the patient arrives, clean the room by sending Reiki with symbols to the walls, the ceiling, the floor and the corners. Burn an incense stick or two. Play soft, soothing music.

(ii) **Talk to the patient:** Listen empathetically to the patient to learn about his or her problem(s). Refuse to treat emergencies, as these fall outside the scope of Reiki (though you can give Reiki while taking the patient to the hospital). Explain the essentials of Reiki in brief; avoid going into complex detail. You might tell the patient about some of your experience as a practitioner, taking care not to credit yourself with any cures. Make it very clear that you cannot predict any particular result, as you are not the controller of Reiki but merely its channel. Explain that Reiki will work in the patient's best interests, and that healing might be hindered if the healee is too impatient or too attached to a specific result. The pressure of expectations must be replaced with complete and unswerving trust. Proceed with treatment only when you are sure that the patient has given you permission and is willing to pay for Reiki with some kind of energy exchange. Politely refuse those who are obviously trying to put Reiki to test and/or prove it ineffective.

(iii) **Prepare yourself:** Wash your hands before (and after) the treatment and avoid using perfume or strong after-shave, as these might trigger an allergic response in your patient. Mentally assume the attitude of gratitude: feel thankful for the opportunity to heal this person. Feel this person to be a mere extension of yourself, so you do not feel superior to him or her in any way. Pray for all the healing powers of the universe, all the teachers of the universe and all the Reiki masters of past, present and future to be with you to guide and bless the healing you are about to undertake. Pray also for your and the patient's spirit guides to be present. Place yourself in a comfortable posture and make sure you are in a relaxed frame of mind, as expressed by your hands and shoulders. It usually helps to have the patient lie on a diwan while you sit on a cushion with your hands at the patient's body level.

(iv) **Prepare the patient:** Ask the patient to remove his or her belt, wallet, wristwatch, rings and other accessories. There is no need to remove the clothing; Reiki can flow through even plaster casts. Have the patient lie down on his or her back with palms up and legs uncrossed. Ask him or her to close his or her eyes and assume an attitude of gratitude for Reiki for agreeing to flow into him or her and provide the necessary healing. Suggest that the patient go totally loose and limp, focus on the bodily sensations that spring up around your hands, be aware of the feelings and thoughts that arise in his or her mind and let such feelings come and go without any suppression or condemnation.

Mentally draw the three Reiki symbols on the patient's crown chakra, and visualize them sliding down to his heart chakra.

(v) **Protect yourself:** To ensure any protection that you might need, draw a big power symbol starting from the top of your head and extending down to your solar plexus. Draw the power symbol with a finger on each of your palms.

(vi) **Comb the aura:** This procedure helps make the patient's aura more receptive. Have your patient stand in front of you at arm's length. Extend your arms above his or her forehead, keeping your hands together but with your fingers spread wide. Imagine your fingers to be extending about half a foot into your patient's body, and mentally comb down the body with your fingers in one single sweep. Do not stop anywhere along the body. When you approach the feet, pull your hands away in a curving motion. Come back to the top of the head and sweep down again, but this time cover a strip just adjacent to the one you just completed. Continue clockwise around the body until you come back to where you started. Do not leave any area uncombed.

(vii) **Scan the body:** See above.

(viii) **Balance the chakras:** See above.

(ix) **Smooth the aura:** See above.

You may choose to skip chakra balancing and smoothing of aura at this stage, and perform them after the completion of full-body Reiki instead.

(x) **Say a Reiki prayer:** A Reiki practitioner normally starts a healing session by closing the eyes, putting hands to chest and then to forehead and bowing the head while mentally saying a prayer. In essence, this prayer should say, 'I am grateful to myself for being here. I am grateful to Reiki for being here. I am grateful to [the patient] for being here.' Your prayer may change as you evolve spiritually; for example, I add the following: 'I surrender completely and pray to Reiki to heal [the patient] complete and whole.'

The prayer is an occasion to remind yourself that:

1. It is not you but Reiki that heals. Alhough you can channel Reiki, you do not have any control over the healing process and cannot predict how Reiki will work.
2. You should not make yourself feel any more valuable, righteous or pure than the patient simply because you are the provider. Each of us has weak points, even if those of the receiver of Reiki are more apparent at this moment.
3. You should feel truly grateful to Reiki for being unconditionally available to you whenever you need it.

(xi) **Begin the healing session:** Become aware of the patient's breathing, and synchronise yours with his or hers. Send your patient love, bliss, positive thoughts, affirmations and good wishes. The patient does feel the difference between a practitioner who is 'with' Reiki and one who is providing it absent-mindedly.

Normally a full-body treatment includes three to five minutes of Reiki at each of the twenty-eight hand positions, but there are no hard and fast rules. You can buy three-minute music tapes to keep you on track, but it's best not to be guided by them even if you play one during treatment. If you pay attention to the sensations, you will know when to shift to the next position; a dissipation of sensation or a patient's deep sigh of satisfaction tell you to move on. Occasionally you may need to hold a position longer, even up to twenty or twenty-five minutes, if it clearly needs more Reiki. Finally, after the full-body treatment you may wish to give extra Reiki to weaker organs, such as the pancreas for diabetic patients or a stiff shoulder or neck. You can never overcharge anyone with Reiki, as it has its own intelligence. When an organ has received enough, Reiki usually diverts itself to other areas where it might be required.

Do not hesitate to give Reiki treatments for want of time. Something is better than nothing. Too little Reiki may be of limited use in some cases, but minor ailments such as headaches, bee stings, toothaches and cuts can often be healed with very little Reiki. If you do not have time for full-body Reiki but want the best possible results, try the following:

Positions for quick treatment:

1. Both hands at the crown chakra.
2. One hand on the forehead, the other at the back.
3. One hand on the front of throat, the other at the back.
4. One hand on the front of the heart, the other at the back.
5. One hand on·the front of the solar plexus, the other at the back.
6. One hand on the front of the hara, the the other at the back.
7. One hand on the front of the genitals, and the other at the back.
8. One hand under the left sole, the other under the right.

Alternately, if you have even less time, use only the foot positions (16-21).

When changing positions, do not move both hands together; always keep one hand on the present position while moving the other to the next. Once the second hand is on the next position, bring the first hand along to join it. Do not exert pressure; the patient should only feel the loving touch and the warmth of your hands. Take special care when your hands are on the patient's eyes and nose; do not obstruct the nostrils.

For specific ailments, hold your hands on the organ involved, and stay there if you find that Reiki is flowing therein. (Your patient can help you confirm this.) If your intuition guides you to another place, follow it and provide Reiki there. Trust your intuition, even if it does not initially seem to work for you—it will start to work better if you trust it. Eventually Reiki may guide you to skip a position or two, or add a new one.

Remember to draw the symbols as advised by your master: the master symbol (if applicable), distant healing symbol, mental/emotional healing symbol and power symbol. Continue with the power symbol only—imagine drawing it deep within those organs that require special attention.

(xii) Spiral: Once you have given Reiki to both feet, you have finished all the positions on the front of the body. You may have to ask the patient to turn around so you can attend to positions on the back of the body, i.e., the D positions. At this point you may need to do a procedure called spiralling to connect the Reiki energy given on the front of body to the energy you're about to give on the back.

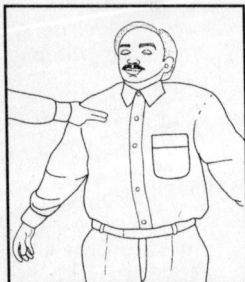

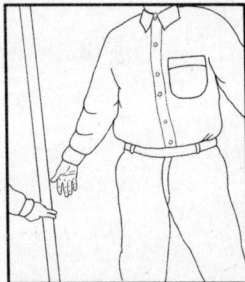

To spiral, locate the triangular notch on the front of the right chest-shoulder joint. Place your index and middle finger at this joint and make a quick, counter-clockwise spiralling movement down the right arm towards the hand. Make a gesture of throwing out the energy (which you have just carried from the joint) over the patient's hand. Now repeat this movement, starting in the same notch but moving along the side of the torso and down the legs towards the feet. Finish with a 'throw-out' gesture at the tip of the right foot. Repeat both movements along the left side of the body.

Ask the patient to turn on to his or her stomach and resume the full-body Reiki session with the back positions.

Note that you cannot perform spiralling on yourself.

(xiii) Sweep: When you have finished full-body Reiki, let the patient lie on his or her stomach and firmly hold your index and middle fingers at the sides of your patient's spine (the base

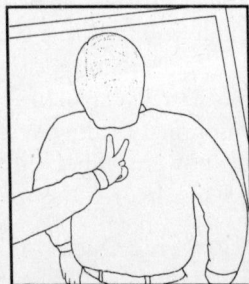

of the throat chakra) and let them sweep down along the spine to the tailbone in one quick stroke. Do not for a moment lose touch with the patient's body or lessen the pressure. (If the patient is diabetic, the stroke should go in the opposite direction, from the tailbone to the throat chakra.)

(xiv) Smooth the aura: See above.

(xv) Beam: Step back from your patient to a distance of about six feet. Imagine powerful, laser-like beams of milky-white Reiki energy emanating from your heart, solar plexus and palms and enveloping your patient's entire body. Imagine that you can direct these beams by moving your eyes. Draw the Reiki symbols in order on the cloud of white light that now surrounds your patient, and linger on the power symbol for a while. Use your eyes to direct the Reiki beam towards any particular organ or part of your patient's body. To improve the efficacy of the beaming process, stay in touch with the Reiki consciousness by riveting your attention on the sensations and feelings you experience with each passing moment.

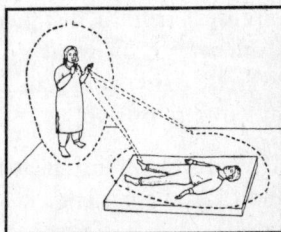

(xvi) Seal the healing: Mentally draw a power symbol on the patient's solar-plexus chakra under the protection of your hands. Pray to Reiki to seal the healing you have just provided with Reiki's love and wisdom. Finish with a loving touch all over the patient's body.

(xvii) Say a closing prayer: 'With the love, mercy and permission of Reiki I declare [the patient]'s life healed, at all levels, complete and whole. Thank you, Reiki. Thy will be done.'

Wash your hands and send Reiki to all sides and corners of the room.

INTERPRETING THE SENSATIONS THAT ARISE

While providing Reiki to others, we often encounter sensations that can point us towards a specific kind of problem or disturbance in the patient's energy field. Though sensitivity to the energy field improves with practice, you can hasten the process. Rub your hands together vigorously for thirty seconds, and bring them together very, very slowly (over about five minutes) from a distance of about a foot-and-a-half apart. Concentrate on what your hands are feeling. If you do this exercise daily, your hands should become reasonably sensitive in a month or two.

Warmth or **intense heat** is the most common sensation. This indicates the patient's need for vitality.

Tingling is often associated with some kind of inflammation. The intensity of the tingling suggests whether the inflammation is chronic, acute or minor. If the tingling is very severe, you might refer the patient to a qualified medical practitioner with a suggestion to find out his or her ESR (Erithrocyte Sedimentation Rate, a test that indicates the possible presence of infection).

Coldness stems from a hidden or forgotten psychological pain that will not allow the organ in question to participate freely in the energy interactions now taking place in the body. The patient should be encouraged to remember, and connect him- or herself to, the scars related to this organ in order to release these energy blocks. Full-body Reiki with an emphasis on this organ should bring the 'disinterested player' on the team back to the game with new enthusiasm, but the patient may need to do a lot of internal work to this end.

Such energy blocks can also be dissolved by imagining that the energy from the block is released and gathers into a ball at the surface of the skin. Imagine that you then hold this ball in your left hand and make a slicing motion with your right hand so as to sever the ball from the skin. Lift the right hand and bring it near the left hand. Imagine that your right hand is shooting out laser-like beams of dazzling white light on to the ball and enveloping it. Imagine the ball being completely dissolved in this dazzling white light and moving up into the air.

Another way to dissolve energy blocks is to pray or call out, 'Father, mother, God, please furnish a fire ball,' and imagine a ball of fire appearing at the side of the patient where the block has been felt. Now imagine yourself pulling tiny energy threads out of the block (as if to disassemble it) and keep throwing them into this fire ball. Imagine the fire consuming them completely. When your intuition tells you the block is gone, pray or call out again, 'Father, mother, God, please take away the fire ball now. Thank you very much.' *Never forget to send the ball away.*

Magnetic repulsion also points towards blocks in the energy field but normally relates to some vital bodily process. The block-release techniques above may help, but the release may take some time.

Magnetic pull indicates the organ's hunger for Reiki energy. Continue giving Reiki to this part of the body until you no longer feel the pull. Before you move on to another part of the body, however, wait and see if any other sensation arises.

Subdued pain is a sign of a block getting ready for release. You may need to channel Reiki to this area frequently until the block is fully released (full-body Reiki may hasten this process). When the released energy rises to the conscious level and is absorbed by the energy field around it, you (and occasionally the patient) feel pointed pain as you come face to face with a repressed player on the body's team. Full-body treatment followed by sincere counselling on the practitioner's part can facilitate the smooth assimilation of whatever energy is released.

The feeling of Reiki flowing through your hands is a welcome sign, indicating that Reiki's love is pouring in and stepping up your vibrational frequency rate.

GROUP REIKI

Group Reiki is an enjoyable experience for both the patient and the channels providing it. Because more than one channel is involved, full-body Reiki takes much less time than a formal one-to-one session. The intensity of healing also gets amplified exponentially, so that Reiki energy provided by four people is not merely four times as strong as that provided by one, but sixteen times that or even more. Practitioners in Dr Hayashi's clinic worked in teams, ensuring that at least two practitioners were available to each patient at any point in time.

My wife, Aruna, and I often provide Reiki to our patients together. Reiki I is the minimum for anyone participating as a practitioner. Both of our children are also second-degree Reiki channels, so on most evenings, one of the four of us receives group Reiki from the other three. This develops a strong bond of love, respect and understanding, not to mention enabling us to share our time in the most meaningful way. Needless to say, it keeps us naturally healthy as well.

The channels begin by holding their hands above the receiver's body, each over their own position. The leader, who attends to the head positions, nods to begin the session and directs it thereafter. While the patient is on his or her back, the leader stays at the shoulders and the person at the feet stays there; the rest of the practitioners cover *alternate* chakras along the spine. For example, one person might attend to the throat and solar-plexus chakras while another puts his or her hands in-between (on the heart and hara chakras). Changes in position are made concurrently, at the leader's direction. If one channel has nowhere to go, he stays at his present position. When the leader is ready to change position (or turn the patient over), he or she checks non-verbally with the others to see if they, too, have finished their part of the healing.

When the session is over, it is the leader's turn to receive Reiki: he or she lies down, and everyone else moves to the position previously held by the channel on their right. This allows every participant to receive Reiki as well as provide it at different positions.

Group Reiki helps channels develop their kinaesthetic sense. Because each channel spends very little time in each position, comparisons in the amount of Reiki drawn by different parts of the body are easily made.

An ideal group treatment has the leader at the head, two people on either side of the torso, one person on each side of the legs and one person at the feet. Any additional channels can sit behind this group and place their hands on the shoulders of someone at one of these positions—thus providing Reiki through, and thereby to, that person. If only two people are present to heal, the one who begins at the head can move to the heart, while the other can begin at the solar plexus and finish at the feet. When the group has three or four channels, the one or two in the middle take care of the torso positions; the other two handle the head and leg (including foot) positions.

The person at the feet may feel the healee's changes in energy intake throughout the session. For example, he or she might feel a slump in the energy when others are giving Reiki to positions with blocks, or a rise in the energy when a healer reaches a new position that starts drawing energy like a thirsty horse drinking from a pond. This channel may also receive intuitive signals about the patient's past and present life situations, and pieces of much-needed guidance. To let the energy move more freely, he or she should keep his or her body out of the range of the energy being released from the patient's feet. Soothing background music can help keep everyone in a quiet, relaxed frame of mind; conversation is best left for another time.

In addition to healing individuals, group Reiki can be used to heal Mother Earth, holes in the ozone layer and damage from an earthquake, flood, famine, cyclone, riot or war. Mother Earth nourishes us throughout our lives and asks for nothing in return; rather than take everything for granted, we can take an opportunity to express our gratitude by sending group Reiki to her.

It is a fine idea to seek out Reiki practitioners in your locality and arrange get-togethers or even Reiki dinner parties, where Reiki can be provided to anyone who needs it or wants to 'taste' it. (Of course, it should be made very clear to those joining the group only as recipients that Reiki requires energy exchange; free Reiki can be given only once or twice.) Such gatherings can begin with group Reiki to Mother Earth or to a common cause that ensures the good of all, and then proceed to the healing of participants. Conversation should be postponed until dinnertime, when participants can share their Reiki experiences. When planning the evening, take care not to delay dinner, as this may be annoying or inconvenient to some.

Group Reiki can also be performed long-distance. The group sits in a circle and imagines the patient to be at the center. Everyone in the group draws the distant-Reiki symbol and then chants the symbol's name three times before sending Reiki by the 'short' method of distance or absentee healing. When the group members themselves are not all in one place, they can start giving Reiki at the same time, preferably imagining themselves gathered together around their patient.

THE NEED FOR ENERGY EXCHANGE

A great deal of well-meant but unnecessary criticism has been levelled at the fees practitioners charge for Reiki attunements and healing sessions. People providing Reiki free of charge are mushrooming all over the world—they believe that humanity needs Reiki more than ever before, so Reiki should be easily available to everyone who wants it. I remember sharing this concern when I was toying with the idea of learning Reiki: I thought I would use it as social work. Charging money seemed contrary to the spirit of service to humanity.

As I grew with Reiki, however, the hollowness of most of my seemingly lofty beliefs was revealed. I realized that the world is already perfect, including all its imperfections, and does not need social workers to make it more perfect. There is no one world! The earth that we share may be one, but there are as many worlds as there are people on this planet, which is why one person feels like commiting suicide while another one is intoxicated by the beauty of life. One makes one's own world through one's attitude, thoughts and responses, and carries this world in one's own mind and heart. Just as you cannot eat the right foods to make someone else healthy, you cannot change another person's world; he or she must bring about the necessary spiritual growth and transformation as a result of his or her own thoughts and deeds.

When Jiddu Krishnamurti, the famous thinker, was asked about his contributions to humanity and world peace through his sixty years of discourses all over the world, he refused to claim any. When asked why, then, he had spent his entire life lecturing, he replied that it was a choice-less choice, just as it is in the nature of flowers to bloom, the birds to fly and sing and the moon to appear beautifully in the sky every night. The only world you need to heal and can heal is your own; spiritual growth cannot be given as alms. If it is not earned, it will get lost as easily as it comes.

Fruitful, mutually satisfying interactions take place on material, emotional, mental and spiritual levels. When you are invited by someone for dinner in response to a great counselling job, the energy exchange is complete: you have enabled him or her to live more peacefully and comfortably, without mental strain, and he or she has saved you the bother of shopping, cooking and serving that meal.

Money and Reiki are both energies. They come from the same source. Just as Reiki is not your energy—it only flows through you when you want it to—money is not the patient's own energy; it simply flows through her when she feels committed to exchanging it. Energy exchange makes the cycle complete in the interest of both parties. Money, like Reiki, is the result of commitment. Once you commit to give money (or anything else) in exchange for Reiki (or anything else), the universe arranges it for you.

Thus, when you say you cannot afford it, you block this flow of energy. The thought that you cannot afford it stems from a scarcity-consciousness which nurtures the illusion that your money is yours, you created it with your hard work, it is finite and you own it. Yet no one can own money—one can only use money so long as one is alive. Money is a mere material reflection of one's inner richness and prosperity-consciousness: you amass it in proportion to the extent of your belief that you deserve it because you belong to the infinitely rich universe. Once you make a commitment to purchase an expensive item, money materializes to enable you to do so—and materializes that much more easily if the item is in harmony with your life purpose and the grand plan of the universe.

In response to hearing all this, people are often quick to ask, 'But what about the poor, who do not have *any* money?' In keeping with the spirit and principles of the universe, genuinely serious and committed people cannot be kept out of Reiki for want of money. Money follows commitment automatically, not the other way around. If someone is committed to Reiki, it becomes the responsibility of Reiki to arrange the necessary funds, or to find a practitioner who will agree to give the necessary discount for anyone who shows real commitment. In rare cases, for some karmic reason, Reiki may want a little more trust and may ask you to spend first, in the knowledge that the money will flow back to you later. The trust that Reiki fulfills this responsibility perfectly has never, to my knowledge, been thwarted. I believe that that the poorest of the poor *can* afford Reiki treatments if only they feel enough hunger to do so and believe it is possible for them to do so.

When I came to Reiki, I had never spent money to learn anything of the kind, and was naturally reluctant to part with my cash in this way. But I found that when I made the decision, I grew a little more detached from my money. With this detachment the problem of money eased, and I never again had to think twice about money for anything related to my spiritual growth. The more you try to hold on to money, the more you impede its flow into your life. The source of Reiki and money is the same—both come to us in response to our resolve, and both can only be used for our happiness. Do not ask God for money; it is abstract. Ask for what you want, and money will be provided for it.

The rates for attunements and Reiki healing sessions vary

from teacher to teacher, but within a narrow range. In exceptional cases, one teacher may decide at his or her own discretion to charge less or more depending on the patient. Reiki treatments may usually cost Rs 50 to Rs 150 per sitting. Attunement seminars cost between Rs 500 to Rs 1,200 at the first level, significantly more at the higher levels. The idea is that someone who comes to get healed or to learn Reiki must feel that he or she is giving slightly more than what is easily affordable.

Energy exchange saves both the patient and the healer from nursing the negative feeling that is likely to arise eventually: namely, that the former is a drain on the latter's time and energy. Needless to say, such negative feelings are detrimental to both and run counter to the spirit of Reiki, which asks us to love and respect every living being (including ourselves). Energy exchange keeps the healer and the patient on the same footing, fostering the feeling of equality.

Often people ask, 'Isn't it too costly?' But I ask in return, 'Costly compared to what?' Reiki seems costly only to those who have not experienced it. Those who pay the fee soon find Reiki to be the best investment they have ever made. The benefits of all the things on which we normally don't mind spending a comparable amount (e.g., trousers, a visit to the beauty parlour, lunch in a restaurant, a tie or some fancy shoes) do not even compare with the permanent blissful transformation that anyone with ordinary sincerity and commitment will inevitably experience in the wake of a Reiki attunement and regular Reiki sessions. Investments in physical things have limited value, as these objects wither with time. It is only our spiritual development that we can take with us throughout our lives, and even when we leave this world behind.

Principles of Healing

Reiki's efficacy is mostly independent of the receiver's conscious will or faith. People do draw Reiki in different intensities depending upon their subconscious willingness or reluctance to be healed, but it is extremely rare to find someone who draws no Reiki at all. It is true that there may be 'cold' parts of the body where Reiki cannot initially gain access because of blockages therein; the speed and efficacy of healing also depend on the extent to which an illness or disease is ingrained in one's energy body.

Reiki's efficacy depends upon the extent to which the patient discloses him- or herself to the healer. The same is true even for self-healing. Most of us fear being admonished or rejected by our 'adult' or logical self (the third kosha), but the journey of healing begins with a ruthless acceptance of what we are, with all our weaknesses as well as strengths. A pre-requisite to cleanliness is acceptance of the fact that there is dirt .

The laws of healing almost always cooperate with the laws of Nature. Reiki may not be able to grow lost limbs for you, but it may work on the other organs and systems and may bring about an indirect positive effect by protecting other organs from the adverse effects that ensue when an organ has been lost or damaged.

Healing takes place in stages. Coming face to face with the problems within—problems that can both surprise and embarrass us—we can find ourselves fluctuating between joy, hope and the will to improve and the frustration of confronting our newly visible weaknesses. Just when you think you have almost healed a particular body part or habit, some other embarrassing ailment or habit surfaces, revealing (in Reiki's wisdom) a series of causes and effects. But every time you deal with a new weakness, you grow stronger and more confident.

For example, someone struggling to get over a drinking habit might find his personal relationships getting uncomfortable. As this draws his attention towards working on relationships, he realizes he has been using alcohol to run away from relationships, and that the relationships were bad because he has been taken for granted—not getting the respect, love or consideration he thinks he deserves. An intuitive thought throws light on his childhood, during which he was forever scolded and humiliated by his parents, siblings and teachers, and how being the youngest in the family made everything he did seem childish. The child within him continues to expect this, and to this day feels most at home when treated this way. Starting with self-affirmation and forgiveness exercises, such a person might find that alcohol addiction has rapidly become a thing of the past and that people have started treating him with respect, love and admiration. Thus, the second stage of treatment results in the gradual dropping away of undesirable attitudes, habits and weaknesses.

At the physical level, the initial turn of events may be for the worse. Because healing focuses a great deal of energy on ailing areas that have thus far been energy-deficient, any pain, suffering and discomfort are felt with greater intensity. The unfortunate result is that many patients stop Reiki at this point, giving up on a healing process that has clearly already begun. As more energy is brought to this area, it dissolves the affliction; the surrounding organs are activated into contributing better to overall health; and the person gets back on the journey towards harmonious balance.

Healing accelerates when the patient takes responsibility for both his ailment and his recovery. The patient should accept weaknesses and deficiencies as they surface, look for the hidden messages they convey, and address them with necessary action. Healing cannot be left solely to extraneous means (including allopathic medicine), for it is essentially an inner process. This is why people with positive attitudes get better faster—the resulting self-discipline leads them to exercise regularly, eat wisely, drink better water, nourish their souls with meditation and other spiritual exercises, release their pent-up feelings and engage in detoxification or other purifying processes. If the patient is willing to give all it takes to get cured, healing is invariably faster and more effective. After all, the universe's purpose in blessing us with illness is to help us learn lessons and grow spiritually in the process.

Healing depends upon the patient's real intentions and perceptions of illness. No one can be cured who perceives illness as a means to higher rewards—attention, love, care, sympathy and lighter responsibilities. Healing does not take place when you do not want it to take place, perhaps because you are not open to it, you want to prove it wrong or you feel challenged by some form of healing because it threatens your long-held beliefs. Similarly, if you perceive your ailment as part of your misfortune, unworthiness or divine punishment rather than part of the universe's wise and natural mechanism for personal growth, there is little chance of being fully cured.

Anything we grow attached to achieving becomes that much more difficult to achieve. Healing becomes difficult when the healer, the patient or both grow too attached to curing a particular ailment. Their focus shifts from learning the intended lessons to merely getting rid of the symptoms, just as you interfere with the sprouting of a seed if you dig up the soil every other hour to check on its progress.

Healing takes place at all levels of being and is reflected in various different aspects of life. People often take healing to mean relief from unpleasant physical symptoms, but symptoms only reflect issues that have yet to be integrated into our lives, or ways in which we are not living as our real, unique selves. So when healing takes place, it may bring changes not only in the physical body but also in other facets of life, such as profession, residence, economic status, creativity and relationships (with others, with oneself and even with inanimate things).

COMBINING REIKI WITH OTHER HEALING METHODS

Reiki can be used in conjuction with any other bona fide therapy, such as allopathy, homeopathy or ayurveda, and indeed it enhances their beneficial effects. It has been shown that the side effects of allopathic drugs can be reduced and even neutralized when treatment is accompanied by Reiki. With the approval of a physician, medicine can eventually be ingested in smaller doses if taken soon after a Reiki session, depending upon the duration and intensity of the session. Reiki obviates altogether the need for pharmaceutical drugs for minor pains, headaches, minor wounds, insect bites and sensitive teeth. However, Reiki does not reduce the effect of painkillers that act on the whole body.

In particular, Reiki mitigates the painful side effects of chemotherapy, which alters the healthy functioning of normal cells while it kills off the harmful ones. Along with its own residue, chemotherapy leaves the residues of the tissues it kills, and these appear on the auric level as dirty, greenish-brown viscous bioplasma. This substance can remain stagnant in the auric field for up to fifteen years, interfering with the natural functioning of the energy field. Parts of the auric field may get burnt or get damaged due to radiation treatments; the immune system is weakened; and the liver gets overburdened with waste. All these things together bring the 'chemo' patient great discomfort. Reiki has been found to dislodge this waste and repair the damaged parts of the aura, not to mention mitigate the patient's suffering and hasten recovery. Only one caveat: Reiki should not be given or sent *during* the chemo sessions themselves.

Because Reiki enhances the body's responsiveness, it also supports homeopathy and other systems that work on the energy level, such as Bach flower essences. When supported by Reiki, homeopathic treatment may be required in progressively smaller doses of higher potencies, and may move from animal resources to mineral and metallic ones. Symptoms also improve in clarity.

REIKI AND DIET

Most of our eating habits are habitual. We tend to take our diet for granted, eating whatever is available or whatever our tongue dictates. Most of us never wonder what our body actually *needs*. Ask yourself for intuitive answers through meditation, and keep your body vibrantly healthy so as to maximize your efficacy as a Reiki channel.

Water. Drinking lots of water helps keep your body free of toxins and wastes. Begin your day with six glasses of water, definitely clean and preferably hot. (You can start with three glasses and gradually increase to six if you find six onerous.) Drink a total of ten to twelve glasses of water every day, skewed towards the morning and afternoon rather than evening. Do not drink cold water, as it cools down the digestive fire (warm water tones the digestive system). Avoid drinking water during a meal; stop forty-five minutes before the meal and wait two-and-a-half hours afterwards before resuming. Dr Deepak Chopra recommends carrying hot water in an insulated flask and taking one or two sips every half hour to keep toxic residues from accumulating in the body. You can enrich the water by magnetizing it or/and giving it Reiki for five minutes. You may also want to take two capsules or tablets of Spirulina with water before breakfast.

Timing. Establish regular mealtimes. Imagine your digestive capacity to be in proportion to the intensity of sunlight at that time.

Breakfast (as late as possible before you leave for work): Breakfast should be light but rich in nutrition. It might consist of freshly drawn fruit juice, dalia, low-fat milk, cottage cheese, cooked oatmeal, lassi, raisin and cinnamon. Don't even think about heavy stuff like fried eggs, buttered toast, pastries or paranthas.

Lunch (ideally at noon, definitely before two o'clock): Lunch can be a little heavier than breakfast, but you should decrease your intake thereafter. Eat the bulk of the day's food by two o'clock. Do not reheat food. If you need to carry your lunch, keep it in a double-walled lunch box so it does not lose its heat by afternoon. Raw foods need a very powerful digestive system, and are best taken as the first course of lunch — your digestive system is as it peak around noon. Unless they are grown organically, fruits or vegetables are usually sprinkled with insecticides and pesticides, so be sure to wash raw foods before you eat them. Salads can include fresh leafy vegetables, cucumbers, carrots, beets and tomatoes, garnished with coriander or mint leaves plus germinated grams. When you begin your main course after the salad, take the protein first (low-fat yogurt, nuts, lentils, peas, beans and soybeans) and then the carbohydrates. Take very little fat.

Dinner (between 6 and 7 p.m.): Dinner should be your lightest meal if you do not want to put on weight. For a good night's sleep, eat more carbohydrates and less protein. Avoid raw foods, especially if your digestion is weak; cooking drives out the toxins. You should ideally have dessert before dinner, but if you still feel like eating something sweet after dinner, go for an apple instead of sweets. Ice creams and other cold sweets should be avoided; if you must have ice cream, have it with lunch rather than dinner.

Attitude. Never eat anything while standing; always sit down to eat, even if you're only taking a snack. Take a small quantity in each bite. Close your eyes and think of Mother Earth, who has presented this food for your sustenance, with deep gratitude. Think gratefully of the families of farmers who tended the crops. Thank the plants (or animals) for giving their lives for your sustenance. Think of food as a sacred offering from Mother Earth and from God, given so you can live, and receive it with utmost respect. Do not waste food.

Giving your food three to five minutes of Reiki before you eat it (or serve it to others) will enhance its nutritive value. Even alcohol and tobacco taste different and are less detrimental if you give them Reiki, provided you take them in moderate quantities. After the meal, give Reiki to your stomach for five minutes to aid in digestion and make you feel less tired.

Take your meals in a peaceful environment, perhaps with soft music, and chew your food slowly and well, especially the first morsel. Avoid talking while eating. Take the next morsel only after you have chewed the present one completely. Pay constant attention to the taste of the food. Do not eat absent-mindedly or in haste; if you are disturbed or angry, it's better to skip the meal.

Quantity. Generally speaking, eat less. This ensures long life. Keep one-fourth of your stomach empty at every meal—prepare only three-fourths of what you normally eat, so that you stop eating when you feel you could still eat thirty per cent more. (That is, if you normally feel full after four chapatis, eat only three.) Do not begin another meal until the previous one is digested—which is to say, do not snack between the major meals, within two to four hours of a small meal and four to six hours of a major meal.

Quality. Make fruits (or their fresh juice), sprouts, salads and green vegetables a major part of your diet. Minimize your intake of dairy products. Humans need very little protein, but many of us consume too much of it, and excess protein results in the accumulation of toxins and acid. Avoid non-vegetarian foods, especially pork. Be a vegetarian not necessarily for love of animals but for love of yourself. Be kind to your body by keeping meat out.

Avoid:

- alcohol
- ice-cold foods and drinks
- white sugar (replace it with gur or brown, unrefined powdered sugar or honey)
- white salt (replace it with black or rock salt)
- polished rice (replace it with unpolished rice)
- maida or white flour (replace it with whole-wheat flour, which is ground with its husk)
- refined or hydrogenated oil (replace it with til oil, if possible)
- Vanaspati ghee (replace it with the kind that has polyunsaturated fats) and butter (replace it with clarified butter)
- tinned foods
- colas
- chocolate
- coffee and tea
- Pasteurized, homogenized or highly heated milk or its products

Use curd instead of milk, except perhaps with cereal. If you do have milk, boil it with turmeric or ginger, adding a little honey when it cools down if you want to sweeten it. Also cut down on onions and garlic (unless you use them for therapeutic reasons), mushrooms and potatoes, as these deplete one's energy.

Seek out organic food and stick to it if possible. It saves our environment as well as our health.

Proportion. Increase your intake of sprouts (if they suit you) as they provide vitamins, minerals and enzymes without straining your digestive system. Combined with nuts (say, fifty grams of groundnuts or khazoor), fresh fruits and vegetables (which may include roots and tubers but must comprise a rich dose of green leafy items), sprouts should make up one-third of your total intake during the day. Apart from being highly nutritious, sprouts are easily digested. The second third should comprise lightly steamed or lightly fried vegetables, and the final third should comprise properly cooked regular foods such as whole-wheat bread (preferably fortified with ragi, bajra or millets, as in roti), corn flakes, soya products or yogurt.

Mixture. Combine your foods intelligently. Do not mix cheese with bread, milk with cereal or rice with pulses. Rice, bread and potatoes are starchy foods that need an alkaline digestive environment, whereas meat, dairy, nuts and legumes are proteins and need an acidic environment. When you mix one kind of food with another, the juices produced by the body neutralize each other and digestion becomes difficult, sapping away a chunk of your energy. The undigested food results in the accumulation of all kinds of toxins and bacteria. Avoid eating different kinds of fruits together, and do not mix fruit with any other foods, especially proteins.

Digestion. Make sure you do some physical exercise each morning, such as walking, yoga, swimming or tai chi. Sit in vajrasana or any other comfortable posture and give Reiki to your stomach. To ensure that you can fall asleep before 10 p.m.—the latest permissible bedtime—strictly avoid colas after

4.30 p.m. and avoid watching TV or working on the computer after 9 p.m.

Fasting. Once every fortnight, observe a full-day fast during which you consume only liquids: lassi, hot water sweetened with honey, small quantities of milk boiled with ginger, or fresh fruit and vegetable juices.

Alternately, to get rid of the toxins accumulated by excess protein: Eat only ripe pineapples the first day, and only apples the second day. Then eat only pineapples on every tenth day. Follow this schedule for two to three months. Do not consume *any* protein.

To get rid of the toxins accumulated by excess salt (which comes from eating often in restaurants or eating pizza, fried foods, pickles, and non-vegetarian foods): Eat only watermelon for two days. You may have a cup or two of tea or coffee during these two days, but without milk and sugar.

To get rid of the toxins accumulated by excess white flour or sweets (if you are not diabetic): Eat only grapes for two days. You may have a cup or two of tea or coffee, but without milk and sugar.

DO'S AND DON'TS

Reiki should not be thrust upon anyone, even people very close to the channel. Infants and animals have their way of showing disinclination, and if you see such disinclination you should respect it. In the case of your own children, use your discretion. Since you can, of course, send Reiki over a distance without the knowledge of the recipient, it is all the more necessary to refrain from doing so against his or her will. Let your intuition guide you. Reiki should not be given to anyone who is angry, seriously ill or under the influence of alcohol, drugs or any other intoxicants.

Conversely, never give Reiki reluctantly. If you are not in the mood, say so.

Pay close attention to the five principles of Reiki. Every

morning, close your eyes to think about them and resolve to follow them during the day. Throughout the day, be aware of how well you are sticking to your resolve. At night, before you fall asleep, review your day in view of these five principles. What, if anything, kept you from following them? How can you address these impediments tomorrow?

Very weak people should be given Reiki for short durations, initially at the soles of the feet. Only after they regain reasonable strength should they receive longer treatments; a weak body may not be able to handle a strong healing reaction. Reiki should also not be given while a patient is in surgery, as this may wake him or her up from anaesthesia. After the operation, provide Reiki at positions A1, B3, B6, C3, C6 and D7. Unless they are physicians themselves, Reiki practitioners should never give medical advice, no matter how certain or confident they feel about it. Medicines should be reduced or stopped only under the direction of a physician. The patient's physician should always be kept informed about the patient's Reiki treatment, especially if the patient is diabetic. (Continued doses of insulin in unchanged amounts may be more than what may be required, because Reiki usually helps regenerate the pancreas.)

Finally, always remember that you, as a Reiki channel, need to keep your body clean and sacred, like a temple.

4

The Mind-Body Connection: The Emotional Roots of Disease, and Holistic Cures

The universe is one—one energy that manifests itself in a multiplicity of forms. Just as countless kinds of trees are rooted in the same earth, different kinds of people and situations are different forms of the same energy. Our ultimate reality is one energy field, of which we are only manifestations with varying energy-information content. Each of us was made to live out a unique aspect or principle of our lives, and yet many of us suppress or even consciously refuse to do so. When we don't 'play' ourselves consciously from within, Nature 'plays' on us from without.

We are meant to accept life's lessons fully, but when we resist certain experiences or the ways in which our lives are unfolding, we distort our natural frequencies into physical, emotional and psychological energy-blocks. These result in illness and disease. For example, if we repeatedly fail to forgive others, Nature will bring us more and more people and situations that require forgiveness—as if giving us opportunities to learn to do so. Eventually, our individual strings of situations show Nature's incredibly accurate assessment of principles we have already learnt and those we still need to integrate in our lives.

Mounting medical evidence now suggests that the accumulated grudges and anger resulting from acute inability to forgive may encourage the formation of gallstones. Unresolved emotions may give rise to upper- or lower-back problems. Nagging and unrealistically high standards or expectations may emerge as liver or digestive problems. In *Decoding the Secret Language of Your Body*, psychiatrist Dr Martin Rush writes, 'I'm aware that there are those of you who find the notion that your mind can make you sick quite without foundation. A few years ago, I would have said the same thing myself. Still the evidence of the connection between the mind and the body is there and can be seen over and over again. When the connection is acknowledged, the emotions that cause negative body events and illnesses can be expressed in other healthier ways.'

Every time you think a thought or feel a feeling, your brain secretes chemicals called neuropeptides, which get stored in the site corresponding to that aspect of your personality. For instance, the feeling that you are not free to do something you particularly cherish may result in the 'download' of the corresponding neuropeptides in your lungs, which may cause increasing congestion there. Failing to get a promotion you have been 'hungry' for—the way an infant is hungry for milk—may induce a secretion of neuropeptides that makes your stomach contract painfully with hunger. Your body stores all of your emotions and remembers all that you have experienced in your life, good and bad.

For this reason, when you feel extremely sad or happy, your whole body responds likewise with every cell. Most people do not 'notice' positive feelings the way they notice negative ones, but when you are happy, your body is happy to be functioning like a well-oiled machine. Happiness and laughter are tonics—not luxuries, but everyday necessities. However busy you may be, and however important you may consider yourself, you must take some time every day to entertain yourself, enjoy life, whistle a tune, sing a song, play or talk with children, watch cartoons or share jokes, give warm and loving hugs to others as though you will never see them again, spend some time outdoors watching clouds move slowly over a serene blue sky, birds fly beneath them and squirrels chase each other through the trees.

These things cost you nothing, and they are *not* a waste of time. Indulging in pleasant pastimes helps you live very close to what life is for—enjoying it and letting others do the same. Happiness is actually what we all live for, but we get so obsessed with the means to achieve it that we forget the end itself.

Of course, being happy does not mean suppressing or ignoring pain. During unpleasant phases of our lives, we tend not to notice the growing discontent within, but our bodies respond with the symptoms of disease (dis-ease). Noticing and addressing this connection may ease the body's burden of communication, allowing it to heal, relax and function smoothly once again. The symptoms of an ailment ask us to realize and incorporate into our personality those aspects of our being that are crying out for expression. The more severe the repression, the more severe the manifestation of this message in the form of physical illness. So each disease carries a loving message from someone who is constantly watching over us, unconditionally concerned with our growth.

Most of us know when we are extremely happy or sad. However, when our emotions are not extreme (which is usually the case), we are not always aware of them. Childhood conditioning discourages the expression of extreme emotions, as they are not considered socially acceptable. Most of us get so good at suppressing our emotions that eventually we have no idea what we are feeling deep within. Denied cognizance by the conscious mind, our emotions have no choice but to find other ways to express themselves and draw attention: through the body.

If we listen to these messages while they are still whispers, we obviate the need for Nature to pound its drum so violently in our ears. But these whispers are often ignored, simply because we do not train ourselves to recognize them or do not pay them much heed. It's true that they must often be discerned intuitively. For instance, upon leaving your office at the end of the day, you feel your heart contracting and an inexplicable sense of unease coming over you. Instinct tells you to return to your work station, and lo! You find your wallet with cash and credit card lying partially visible beneath a file. Or the phone rings, you pick it up and your wife asks you to proceed directly to your son's school, as he missed the afternoon bus and is waiting patiently for you to pick him up.

If you trust these hunches, you preclude the necessity for guidance to come at a grosser level, wherein the vibrations carrying the message rise to the conscious mind and have a distinctly nervous quality. Alas, however, most people try to push such hunches down into their subconscious by giving in to addictive behaviours such as drinking, overeating, watching endless television and so forth. The message one is supposed to receive starts appearing as an image ('golden idea . . . I can see that happening very clearly'), sound ('that rings a bell for me'), taste ('the meeting left a bitter taste in my mouth') or touch ('we're on a sticky wicket'). At the next stage, the vibrations become recognizable emotions, making you feel disturbed, irritable, heavy or sad. If you find yourself low or irritable, think back over the day's happenings and see if you can track the cause of this uncomfortable emotion. It may stem from a derogatory comment from your boss, your failure to keep a promise to your wife, having done something against your value system, or anything else. Just recognize it and acknowledge to yourself, 'I am feeling upset because I expected him to trust me, since I have never given him or anyone else any reason not to.'

If not acknowledged, the information coded in these vibrations will manifest itself as a headache, shoulder pain, lower-back pain, wrist pain, indigestion or a more deeply entrenched addiction such as pornography or alcohol. Ignoring these signals welcomes them into your daily life, and pushes you towards pain-killers and other kinds of drugs. Eventually you can find yourself with an outright illness or even disease—perhaps a flu that sticks to you for two weeks, an ulcer, a heart attack or cancer. If you do not listen to the inner cries of the soul, you force nature to attract your attention by shouting even more loudly at you—you lose your job, you meet with an accident, someone cheats you of a great deal of money. You may unconsciously invite depression, coma or nervous breakdown just to keep yourself from having to listen to all this.

Good health, therefore, is the reward for being ruthlessly honest in anticipating, acknowledging, accepting and sharing our negative as well as positive emotions, at least to ourselves. This can happen only if we are alert to what is happening in our emotional world. Suppressing emotions not only fails to save us from pain, but it stifles our capacity to experience positive emotions. An emotion, whether strong or feeble, is like an arrow that has been shot—it is *bound* to express itself.

Illness is usually thought of as something we need to fight and ideally, conquer. We invent powerful drugs to 'attack' the illnesses that befall us. In fact, however, illness is like the good but difficult advice of a sincere, well-meaning friend. Instead of listening to the advice, we aim to kill both the message and the messenger. I do not advocate ignoring illnesses and their allopathic cures; I only ask that you understand the message an illness conveys, as the cure lies chiefly in understanding and addressing it. It is true that germs, viruses, bacteria and other micro-organisms cause us many diseases, but they usually manage to harm us only when our resistance to them is low.

To assist you in deciphering the messages that various kinds of disease convey, this chapter outlines the correlations between our emotions and all common physical ailments. Just as dream symbols have different meanings for different people, emotions affect people in different ways, so you may have to do some careful, ruthlessly honest soul searching to track down the lessons uniquely meant for you. Like any other skill, the practice of interpreting these lessons takes constant practice, but it is endlessly interesting and ultimately one of the most rewarding journeys one can undertake.

In addition to delineating the possible mind-body connections for each ailment, I have also indicated the affirmations and attitudinal changes required, the appropriate Reiki positions and the best dietary and natural supplements for lasting holistic healing.

AFFIRMATIONS AND ATTITUDE

Affirmations are short, crisp, powerful statements meant to be repeated to oneself with feeling and conviction about twenty times each, thrice a day—in the morning, during the day and at bedtime.

Affirmation and attitudinal change are key to faster, longer-lasting healing. If you wish, you may occasionally change these affirmations slightly to feel more at home with them or make them more meaningful in your context, but you must always repeat them to yourself with intense conviction. Because the range of negative emotions that cause illness is not vast, I have designed a list of affirmations from which you can select those that apply to your particular problem. You may even decide to repeat the whole list every day, like a prayer, to keep yourself healthy; or you may choose to repeat only the affirmations you find most attractive or most difficult to accept. Difficulty accepting a particular affirmation indicates a corresponding, deeply entrenched negative attitude in that area.

The affirmations can be integrated with Reiki treatments as well. Have the patient write down the result he or she wants to achieve along with the corresponding affirmation(s). Take the paper and draw the mental/emotional symbol on it with your middle finger, then put it in an envelope and seal it. Give the envelope back to the patient and ask him to keep repeating the affirmations mentally throughout the Reiki treatment while holding the envelope in one hand. You should also imagine that you are projecting the affirmations into the person's being. You can use the same envelope in subsequent sessions, but once the intended result manifests itself, bury the envelope in soil.

To develop an attitude of:	Try this affirmation:

Abundance

1. The universe is abundant in all respects. There is an abundance of everything all around us — enough of everything for each one of us, including myself. I encourage this abundance to flow freely into my life by wishing the same for everyone else.

Flexibility

2. I bury the past in the past, and welcome the present with the fresh fragrance of my positive attitude.

3. Going neither faster nor slower than my natural pace will put me in harmony with Nature, and thereby ensure her full support for me in fulfilling my life purpose.

4. I accept the fact that life is change, and I shall therefore readily adapt to every change

5. Whether insult, disappointment, slight or hurt, every experience in my life has come only to teach me something. I am grateful to God for providing me with it and for giving me this opportunity to move ahead in life.

6. I am open to releasing all my fears and my erroneous and limiting beliefs and replacing them with beliefs that empower me with courage and conviction, make me stand straight and tall.

7. I am free—I am the master of my life. I enjoy life because it is meant to be enjoyed. I release my grip on all that I am attached to and I move towards a life permeated with love and relaxation.

8. I hereby forgive everyone against whom I have been carrying a grudge, release all

my resentments towards the world and accept all my experiences unconditionally as the very expression of the most kind God. I begin a new life today, and see it with new and joyous eyes.

9. Every moment, I create from my inner beauty a life that I love to look at.

Freedom

10. Being connected to God has made me rise beyond all my past limitations in mysterious and incredible ways.
(See also Affirmation 7.)

Forgiveness, acceptance of others

11. I allow others the freedom to be who they are, and I accept them as they are.

12. I shall feel no more hate or vengefulness. I choose to open my heart and let limitless love flow out from it in thoughts, words and deeds.

13. I accept and see this person with love, compassion, understanding, joy and gratitude.
(See also Affirmations 5 and 8.)

Gratitude

14. I am grateful for all that I have been blessed with. I thank God for presenting me with this wonderful gift of life, and all that I have received or experienced through it.

15. My body is the temple of the Highest. I maintain its purity to show my reverence for the Highest Power.
(See also Affirmation 5.)

Harmony, perfection

16. I see love, peace and harmony wherever I choose to look, within or without myself. I have surrendered my life to God completely, and that is why I feel eternally secure, safe, protected, loved and nourished wherever I move in time or space.

17. I trust and surrender to the universe, where

every thing is perfect. Since I am a part of the universe, I allow my sexual principles to operate naturally through my body with ease and joy.

Joy

18. I am full of energy. I live life to the hilt.

19. I rejoice in every moment of this life.
(See also Affirmations 7 and 8.)

Love

20. Life is blissful togetherness in family life, created with bonds of love, laughter and empathy. I am so grateful to God for the opportunity to create and rejoice in my family.
(See also Affirmations 7, 12 and 15.)

Wishing happiness for oneself and others

21. Love, joy and happiness for others—these are what I experience and wish, every moment of my life. These are what I have in my heart and these are what I give to others. No wonder these are precisely what come back to me.
(See also Affirmations 8 and 13.)

Relaxation, safety, security

22. Having surrendered my life completely to God, I am deeply relaxed. I know the world is a safe place to live.

23. If God is for us, who can be against us?

24. God's delays are not God's denials. God knows my needs better than I do, and ensures that I get what is right for me when the time is right.

25. I feel so secure, supported and loved because I am an extension of the same Oneness that sustains and nourishes everything.
(See also Affirmations 5, 7 and 16.)

Self-esteem

26. I accept, love, respect and approve myself completely.

27. I am proud of who I am, regardless of what others think of me. What matters is what

I feel about myself.

28. I accept myself unconditionally, with deep love.

29. I am not influenced by statistics or by what others believe. I listen intently to my inner voice, and act on it with trust.
(See also affirmation 7 and 15.)

Self-forgiveness

30. I forgive myself completely, because I did what seemed best at that particular time. It is unfair to judge my past actions with the knowledge and wisdom I possess only now.

Self-expression

31. I express my views and desires freely, with complete trust in the order of the universe.

Trusting myself as a man/woman

32. I am proud to be a complete woman in complete charge of my life. I trust my body fully for the perfect way it works.

33. I am proud to be a complete man in complete charge of my life. I trust my body fully for the perfect way it works.

Understanding, listening, seeing others' points of view, seeing things as they are

34. I know that whatever I hear from others, however unpleasant, is uniquely arranged by God for me and has a purpose. I shall listen intently with love to everything others have to say.

35. I know that life is just an interpretation. Others' perceptions can be just as right for them as mine are for me.

An 'attitude' is a way of responding to the world. Our responses are often subconscious; we realize what we have done only after we have done it. Every night before you go to bed, sit in silence and go through the day's happenings to see if your responses were in line with the desired attitudinal change. If not, think of the response you *should* have produced.

Try the 'Swish' technique to ensure that you respond

differently hereafter. It helps replace deep-rooted negative responses with responses in harmony with the principles of Reiki.

The Swish Technique

1. Sit comfortably erect in a chair and take a few slow, deep breaths.
2. Close your eyes and start picturing vividly the action you want to replace. Think of the colours, sounds and feelings surrounding it. Imagine that you have knobs to adjust colour, volume and even feelings; adjust them all for clarity. Bring yourself into the image. Stay with this image for a while.
3. Let the image shrink suddenly. Then, re-enlarge it to occupy the full screen as a new image of your desired new behaviour. Add colour, sounds and feelings for clarity and vividness. Stay with this image for a while.
4. Do this for a few days, until you start getting results. The effectiveness of the Swish technique depends on how quickly you replace the old image with the new one.

REIKI AND YOUR BODY

Now that you know the Reiki hand positions, you can apply them to specific ailments for faster, more effective healing. Providing Reiki to yourself is recommended if your ailment is chronic; it can also be used simply as a supplement to your treatments with a practitioner.

Unless another duration is mentioned, provide Reiki for at least five minutes, or until you no longer feel the sensations associated with Reiki. Longer durations can never harm, however, and are in fact desirable if you can afford them, especially for chronic diseases. For any ailment, provide Reiki for four consecutive days at the start; then, if the condition improves, you can reduce Reiki to thrice a week and eventually twice a week. If the condition does not improve, you may have to expand to full-body treatment for four days before resuming the shorter treatments in specific positions. If the ailment is chronic, you should keep treatments on a daily basis. If possible, supplement regular treatments with distance healing for better and faster results.

Once you reach Reiki II, provide Reiki to others with symbols. If you can track down a traumatic incident in the patient's life that may have caused his or her ailment, send Reiki with symbols to that incident. Remember: do not be perturbed by any aggravation of symptoms. The more toxins in the body, or the more inner work required, the more severe the healing reaction might be. If the reaction becomes unbearable for the patient, you may decide to increase the interval between two Reiki treatments in order to mitigate the aggravation. If you have any doubts, discuss the healing reaction with a doctor or naturopath, preferably one with some knowledge of Reiki.

Often people wonder whether diseases are caused and cured by the mind or by the diet; it cannot be both. I have personally found that the two are linked: the kind of food we eat affects our thoughts. For each ailment addressed below, I have suggested ways you can use food to to supplement the healing process. These can be modified according to the availability of certain foods; if, for example, out of four dietary suggestions you can follow only one, fine.

Wheat-grass juice is recommended for a great many health problems. To make it, sow a handful of high-quality wheat grains in an earthen pot. Take care of the soil with manure and careful watering. Grass shoots shall grow six to seven inches high in a week's time. Take them out with their roots, wash them and use a juicer to extract the juice, or chem them fresh to drink the juice and spit out the remains. To have juice available every day, you will need seven such pots.

THE BRAIN

The head is our drawing room—our first chance to represent ourselves. Any problem in the head communicates an inner disharmony between who we are and what we have done. Stressful thoughts create rigidity or other problems in the jaws, teeth, neck, shoulders and lower back. Tension can also reach the temples and scalp.

Alzheimer's Disease

Alzheimer's disease is a brain disorder caused by pre-senile brain atrophy: that is, a premature shrinkage of the brain and slowing down of mental processes—bringing premature senility as a result. Alzheimer's disease often begins with forgetfulness and progresses to confusion, irrationality, increased irritability and frustration. Forgetfulness may grow extreme; the patient repeatedly perform actions that have already been performed or ask questions that have already been answered. Metaphysically speaking, Alzheimer's stems from extreme pessimism. Those who attract this disease are angry with the world and refuse to accept it as it is. Through senility, one tends to return to one's childhood (which one found safe and secure) in order to attract attention from others.

Recommended Affirmation: 8

Reiki Positions: Full-body treatment with an extra ten minutes on each head position (A1–A6). If you have time, add B1 and D5.

Dietary and Other Suggestions:

- Drink milk and eat carrots, spinach, green peppers, lettuce, kelp, dark-green leafy vegetables, alfalfa, cabbage, beans, soybeans, potatoes, grapes, grapefruit, lemons, oranges, turnips, onions and garlic.
- Cut down on antacid tablets.
- Give up alcohol.
- Do not cook with aluminium pots or utensils.

Amnesia

Amnesia refers to various kinds of memory loss that may be due to old age, brain injury or a brain disorder. It indicates a deep-seated fear of life, and corresponding unwillingness to face life or speak for oneself.

Recommended Affirmations: 4,18, 22 and 31

Reiki Positions: A1–A6. In addition, provide distance or mental healing to the whole being, with a focus on restoring the memory.

Dietary and Other Suggestions:
- Drink tea prepared with rosemary or dried sage leaves once or twice a day.
- Have an apple with two teaspoons of honey for breakfast.
- Try hypnotherapy under the guidance of an exper hypnotist.

Brain Tumour

Brain tumours represent erroneous beliefs and stubborn negative habits. There is a tendency to hold on to hurts, a refusal to move on and take life as it comes. Trust life and surrender yourself to its flow. The future is precious and needs to be welcomed with the lessons—not scars—of the past.

Recommended Affirmations: 5, 6 and 30
Reiki Positions: A1–A6
Dietary and Other Suggestions: Fast for two days to remove any toxins you may have accumulated from a high-salt, high-sugar or high-protein diet (see 'Reiki and Diet' in Chapter 3). If all three apply, observe the three fasts in succession, with a week between each.

Between fasts:
- Eat more sprouts.
- Heat some powdered black pepper and basil leaves in a glass of water, mix in two teaspoons each of ginger juice and honey, and drink it every morning.
- Mix half a glass each of carrot and beetroot juice and take it thrice a day.
- Avoid exertion.

Cerebral Palsy

Cerebral palsy, a condition of impaired coordination of the limbs, results from a brain injury during pregnancy, birth or early childhood. Hard to detect during infancy, it is often noticed when the child fails to develop the motor abilities expected at each age, such as crawling, walking and self-feeding. The disease shows a need to bring the family together with love.

Recommended Affirmations: 7, 12 and 20
Reiki Positions: A2, A5, B1, B3, B5 and D5

Dietary and Other Suggestions:
- Those suffering from cerebral palsy cannot eat much, so care should be taken to provide them with wholesome, nutritious foods such as porridge, soup and juice. Consult a dietician to devise an appropriate food regimen.

Coma/Narcolepsy

Comas indicate a fear of life, a wish to avoid someone or something altogether. Narcolepsy, which results in fits of sleepiness and drowsiness, stems from a similar escapism, reflecting an inability to cope with life situations.

Recommended Affirmations: These must be used by those attending to the patient rather than by the patient him- or herself. Modify affirmations 7, 16 and 23 to 25 accordingly. For example, you can imagine the patient saying these, or say them yourself using the word 'you' instead of 'I'.

Reiki Positions: A1–A6, B1, B3, B5 and D5 along with group full-body mental healing or intention Reiki for twenty minutes twice or thrice a day.

Epilepsy

Epilepsy involves electrical disturbances in the brain cells, resulting in seizures. The patient may suffer fits of convulsions, then temporarily fall unconscious. Seizures can be triggered by stress, fatigue, excess alcohol, fever and menstruation. They represent the struggle life has become, and the patient's deep desire for revenge.

Recommended Affirmations: 7, 8, 13, 16, 17 and 21

Reiki Positions: A1–A7, B2, B6, D1–D7, the wrists and between the shoulder blades.

Dietary and Other Suggestions:
- Discontinue white salt (replace with rock salt), white sugar (replace with honey or jaggery powder), white flour (replace with whole-grain wheat flour), tea, coffee, cola, smoking and alcohol.
- Cut down on animal proteins (replace with pulses and soybeans) and eat more fresh fruits and vegetables.

- Discontinue foods with additives such as colouring/ flavouring agents and preservatives.
- Do some physical exercise every morning, such as walking, yoga, swimming or tai chi.
- Never overeat.
- Take plenty of vitamin-D milk, millet and cheese.
- Drink several glasses daily of the juices of garlic and of vegetables such as kale, beet tops, spinach, cabbage, lettuce, chard, peas, green beans, carrots and tomatoes.

Forgetfulness

Forgetfulness, common in people over fifty, reflects a refusal to let go of a past unpleasant experience. The purpose of unpleasant experience is to teach us important lessons, which we must use to move on and grow spiritually. People who develop forgetfulness do not learn the necessary lessons from these episodes; they just get stuck in unpleasantness. Their focus is not on solving or learning from problems, but rather on drawing attention and sympathy from others.

The only things you should carry from the past into the future are lessons (not to be confused with prejudices and preconceived notions). Be aware of the conditioning and paradigms through which you perceive the world, and you will experience your present more meaningfully. Live each moment to the fullest; do not let it be contaminated by guilt from the past or worries about the future.

Recommended Affirmations: 2, 5, 6 and 30

Reiki Positions: A1–A6 plus distance or mental healing to the whole being.

Dietary and Other Suggestions:

- Eat an apple, with skin and seeds, a little while before dinner.
- Take five almonds, two carrots, and some aniseeds with a cup of milk every morning.
- Drink a tablespoon of wheat-grass juice once a day.
- Take ten basil leaves, five almonds, and eight grains of black pepper with melted butter and a little bit of jaggery powder once a day.

- Take a mixture of the juices of kale, parsley, red pepper, spinach, asparagus, carrot, cantaloupe and collard greens once a day.
- Give up alcohol.
- Do some mindfulness exercises. To stay in conscious touch with your actions, run a mental commentary on what you are doing at any point in time.
- Learn nadi shodhan and bhastrika pranayama.

Headaches/Migraines

Headaches can strike for many different reasons, and even experts cannot always identify the cause. They often accompany a feeling of guilt for not having behaved or performed as you would have liked. Constant worrying, unreasonable goals and obsession with perfection also contributes to the stress that may cause headaches. Say goodbye to headaches by spending a few days abstaining from judging yourself or the situations in your life. Accept life as it comes.

Migraines involve pounding pain on one side of the head, nausea and sometimes vomiting. Smiling outwardly while suppressing feelings of hate, dislike, anger, guilt or disgust towards yourself or others can cause severe headaches and migraines. Reduce your expectations of both yourself and others. Migraines have a lot to do with resisting the way life unfolds for you, or with suppressing your sexual urges or feeling unnecessarily guilty about them. Seventy per cent of migraine patients are females.

Recommended Affirmations: 7, 16 and 22–26

Reiki Positions: Apart from the top of the head, providing Reiki in the groin region can be helpful. As you feel a migraine approaching, provide yourself with Reiki for ten minutes at each of the following positions. You can skip positions that do not seem to be drawing much Reiki.

- A1–A2, A4–A5 and/or the exact location of the headache
- B2–B3 and B5–B7 (for females, give B7 extra time)
- C2–C3 and C5–C6
- Across the shoulder blades, D1 and D7 (for males, give D7 extra time)

- Wrists

Dietary and Other Suggestions:

- Give up or avoid the following: alcohol, smoking, ice cream, chocolate, coffee, cheese, yogurt, eggs, pork, bacon, ham, Chinese food, all salty foods, sausages, pickles, peanuts, salt, chewing gum, tomatoes, broad beans and citrus fruits.
- To increase your magnesium intake and reduce platelet stickiness, eat lots of garlic, ginger, parsley, carrots, apples, tofu and canteloupe and drink wheat-grass and lemon juice.
- Eat more yeast, whole-wheat bread, nuts and leafy green vegetables.
- Take light meals and keep to your bedtimes, even on holiday.
- Stop drinking milk for about a month and see if it helps.
- Massage the inner side of the big toe, next to the second toe.
- Massage the earlobes with your thumb, middle and index fingers.
- Walk a mile. If the cause of the headache is accumulated gas, it will be released.
- Do yoga, yoga nidra, Sudarshan Kriya and/or meditation to keep your stress level down.
- Squeeze the web between the thumb and index finger, and press the bony ridges at the back of your neck with both thumbs twice a day.
- Avoid aspirin and other pain-relief pills.
- Females prone to migraines should rest with a cold pack under the base of the skull prior to the onset of the menstrual period.
- Sleep on your back or on your left side, with knees bent slightly towards the chest. Use a pillow to ensure that your head is horizontal. Thin, bony people can insert a small pillow between the knees as well.
- Do not overwork.
- Use an anti-glare, anti-radiation screen on your computer screen if you work for long periods. If possible, take an hour-long break after every two hours of computer work.

Insanity

Insanity represents escape from family responsibilities or unpleasant family situations.

Recommended Affirmations: 5

Reiki Positions: A1–A6 plus distance or mental healing to the whole being.

Dietary and Other Suggestions:

- Grind ten black peppercorns with Brahmi leaves and administer them with a cup of water daily, till you feel satisfied with the results.

Mental Diseases

When life becomes too difficult to bear or seems too fruitless to pursue, some people delve into the realm of the unconscious, resulting in conditions like schizophrenia. One must see for oneself the unconscious forces by which one is controlled, and learn to integrate them into one's life.

Recommended Affirmation: 5

Reiki Positions: Five minutes each at B1–B2 and C2–C7. Balance the chakras and provide second-degree Reiki to the head positions to help accelerate the integration process.

Dietary and Other Suggestions:

- Eat plenty of fresh fruits, leafy green vegetables, dried fruits and nuts.
- Take a garlic clove with every major meal.
- Use the colour violet in your clothes and surroundings.
- Practise progressive relaxation with soft, healing music.

Stroke

A stroke is a sudden tapering or loss of consciousness, sensation and voluntary motion caused by the rupture or obstruction of an artery in the brain. It usually occurs when one gives up on life rather than choosing to change oneself.

Recommended Affirmations: 5 and 17

Reiki Positions (for preventive or therapeutic use only, not for emergencies):

- Full-body Reiki twice over, preferably with symbols, for four consecutive days. Give about an hour-and-a-half extra to positions A1–A6, B1, B3, B5 and D6 and any other affected areas. Also give extra time to the body parts directly opposite those affected by the stroke side.

Dietary and Other Suggestions:

- Eat two apples a day and more fruits and vegetables generally, especially pumpkin and lettuce.
- Eat more garlic and take one clove with each meal.
- Avoid pickled foods, salty foods, saturated fats, excess alcohol and meat of any kind. You can have oily fish if it is not salted, pickled or smoked.
- Lose any excess weight.
- Do meditations and yoga nidra.
- Avoid strenuous exercise. Take up a gentler exercise such as swimming, bicycling, brisk walking (not running, but enough to cover a mile in fifteen minutes), yoga or tai chi.
- Visualize, for ten minutes every day, your blood pressure coming down.

THE EARS

Our ears are instruments for hearing what others say. The state of our aural health reflect our openness to doing so.

Deafness/Tinnitus/Earaches

Deafness is an indirect response to something you are constantly being made to hear against your wishes. When you refuse to listen externally, you refuse to listen from within as well—you turn a 'deaf ear' to your inner voice. Deafness forces you to listen to your inner voice, as you can no longer hear anything external. Old age need not distance you from others in this way; staying open and receptive to others helps keep your hearing intact. Earaches are indirect expressions of anger at what you hear externally.

Recommended Affirmations: 5, 8, 12 and 34

Reiki Positions:

- A3 (variation) for fifteen minutes, twice a day.
- A1, A6, B1, C3-C4 and C6-C7 for at least five minutes each.

Dietary and Other Suggestions:

- Fry five cloves in two tablespoons of sesame oil. Filter the oil into a bottle through a clean piece of thin cloth. Soak a little cotton in this oil and place it in the affected ear (or just place two drops in the ear) before going to sleep every night.
- Eat plenty of garlic, onion, chilli pepper and horseradish (to reduce mucous) and whole-wheat bread.
- Cut down on high-saturated-fat foods such as butter, fried foods and red meat.
- In addition, for tinnitus, mix one tablespoon each of dry ginger, jaggery powder and pure ghee and consume it hot.

THE EYES

What is true for the ears is also true for the eyes. Vision problems indicate your reluctance to see something about yourself or your life. The reluctance to see is manifested in blurred vision. Providing Reiki to any disturbing events in your life around the time you began to wear specs—events you would rather not have seen—may help improve your vision. You also need to ask yourself whether there is anything in your current situation that you'd rather not see.

Cataracts are a painless clouding of the eye's lens as a result of oxidation. Metaphysically, cataracts represent pessimism about the future. Vitamin C (found in citrus fruits and gooseberries) and riboflavin (milk, whole-grain cereals and yeast extracts) may help prevent cataracts.

Conjunctivitis, or pink-eye, is the inflammation of the conjunctiva, the eye's delicate outer membrane, as a result of infection or allergy. It indicates inner conflict, anguish and frustration that you have refused to look at consciously. The redness forming a ring around the front of the eye indicates a riboflavin deficiency, while the soreness, redness and cracking at the outer corners of the eyes signal a shortage of B vitamins. Close your eyes, and in the silence that follows, let your inner being whisper this inner conflict to you.

Dry eyes indicate a lack of love and softness in your life.

They draw your attention towards the need to release your anger and forgive.

Twitching eyes represent your inability to look straight into someone's eyes due to fear, nervousness, or lack or loss of self-esteem.

Glaucoma is a condition of increased pressure from the inner ocular fluid. Symptoms include blurred vision, a halo effect around lights, and difficulty seeing in the dark. On a physical level, glaucoma indicates deficiencies of thiamin and vitamin A; on a metaphysical level it indicates that you are unnecessarily but overwhelmingly caught up in pain or grief. Choose to forgive, and give Reiki to the past events that have hurt you.

Itchy eyes suggest that you have repressed a situation—sorrow, disappointment, nostalgia or joy—that would normally have caused you to cry. Tears are being held back at the eyelid.

Keratitis, or inflammation of the cornea, represents extreme anger at what you are seeing, and a desire to hit back.

Myopia hypermetropia and astigmatism, respectively, represent fear of the future and fear of the present.

Astigmatism is a subconscious attempt not to see the self.

Styes are small, red bacterial boils on the glands that lubricate the eyelashes. Recurring styes indicate poor nutrition, stress and/or anger at what one sees in one's life. They can be alleviated with multivitamins and minerals, and brought to a head with a hot compress of cotton wool or a bunch of grated carrots wrapped in a clean cloth.

Recommended Affirmations (for all eye ailments): 4–5, 8–9, 14, 16, 18–19, 21–22, 24–26 and 28

Reiki Positions: A1 for fifteen minutes at least twice a day, depending upon the severity of the problem, and A2, A5, B2, B6–B7, C3, C6 and D2–D7.

Dietary and Other Suggestions:

- Soak trifla (a mixture of harr, bahera and amla) in water in an earthen pot. Filter it through a clean cloth, and rinse your eyes with this water.
- Soak a piece of cotton in some cow's milk and place it over the eye with a bandage before you fall asleep. Remove the

bandage in the morning.

- Palming: Close your eyes and cover them with your palms. Look intently at the ensuing darkness for ten minutes, imagining that it's getting darker and darker.

- Cover your eyes with a handkerchief and tie it at the back of your head. Do this every day for fifteen minutes, or whenever it is possible to rest your eyes. For added benefit, provide Reiki while doing so. Keep your eyes closed while commuting in a car or bus to save them from the ill effects of pollution.

- Eat plenty of nuts, whole grains, citrus fruits, apricots, bananas, mangoes, carrots, sweet potatoes, leafy green vegetables (especially spinach), vegetable juices (especially cauliflower juice) and soups, seed oils and wheat-grass juice, as all these are beneficial to the eyes.

- Soak five almonds in water overnight. In the morning, grind them into a paste and drink it with a cup of milk.

- Mix a tablespoon of dry coconut powder with two tablespoons of jaggery powder and eat it with a little powdered black pepper.

- Massage the soles of your feet with mustard oil at bedtime.

- Keep the light on while watching television. Cover the top of the VDU with black cartridge paper, folding the sides down over the sides of the VDU. Tune down the VDU's brightness and adjust the contrast as necessary. Use an anti-glare, anti-radiation computer screen if you work for long durations, and take an hour-long break every two hours if possible. Palm your eyes for one minute after every ten minutes of work before a VDU. Take short, frequent breaks from work to close your eyes for a few seconds.

- Get as much sleep as your body needs, whether it's seven hours, nine hours or more. No remedy will work if you are not getting enough rest.

- Keep your eyes closed when you are not required to use them (while commuting, on the phone, listening to music, sitting through commercials on television). Blink more often—at least once every three minutes.

- Boil some eye-bright tea and soak a towel in it after it has cooled a bit. Hold the warm towel over your eyes for fifteen minutes, taking care that no tea actually enters your eyes. Bright-eye tea can be had from any chemist.
- Never read in a moving vehicle. 'Time management' at the cost of the health of your eyes is not a good prescription.
- Do not exceed any prescribed dose of eye drops.

THE MOUTH

The mouth represents our ability to take in new ideas and information, and act on new impulses. Oral complaints show difficulties in this area; for example, a yawn represents dislike or boredom.

Adenoids

An adenoid is an enlarged mass of lymphatic tissue between the back of the nose and the throat (above the tonsils), caused by repeated infections or allergies. It usually occurs in children, and manifests itself in difficulty breathing or speaking. Adenoids indicate that the parents or elders have not accepted the child completely. Parents must understand that children are not their behaviour; imperfection is part of Nature's perfection. Each of us has come to this earth because we have something to learn, including the child in question. Accept him as he is—this will encourage him to learn what you want him to learn.

Recommended Affirmations: 13
Reiki Positions: A1, A3, A5–A7 for five to seven minutes each.
Dietary and Other Suggestions:

- Keep an ionizer in the child's bedroom at night to remove any nasal congestion.
- Add a few drops of mustard oil to the child's hot bathwater.
- Increase the child's resistance to infection by introducing a diet rich in citrus fruits, leafy green vegetables, onions, tomatoes, potatoes, sweet potatoes and garlic.
- Cut down on dairy products until the adenoid is healed. In place of milk, give the child soya milk.

- Thrice a day, pour a cup of boiling water onto two or three teaspoons of goosegrass (also known as clivers or cleavers), leave it undisturbed for fifteen minutes and then eat it.

Bad Breath

Bad breath can simply be the result of eating spicy food, onion or garlic, but it can also indicate an infection, a tooth or gum disorder, a zinc deficiency, a gastrointestinal problem (that emits gases and odours) or even syphilis. Persistent bad breath indicates persistent unpleasant thoughts (such as anger or revenge) that need cleansing. Tell yourself several times each day that you are releasing the past with love.

Recommended Affirmations: 4–8, 10, 16, 19 and 21
Reiki Positions: A1–A2, A5–A7, B2–B7 (with emphasis on B2 and B6) and D5 for five to seven minutes each.
Dietary and Other Suggestions:

- Rinse your mouth with a glass of water mixed with a few drops of lemon or ginger juice.
- Eat roasted caraway grains, and chew cloves and parsley.
- Chew coriander and basil leaves.
- Eat plenty of apples and raw vegetables for healthy gums; ginger, cinnamon, mustard and horseradish for healthy sinuses; whole-grain cereals and water to avoid constipation; carrots, broccoli and spinach for beta carotene; and citrus fruits and gooseberry for vitamin C.
- Avoid garlic, onions, alcohol and tobacco. Cut down on cakes, biscuits and other sugary foods.
- Use a tongue cleaner every morning and evening.

Dry Mouth

A complete lack of saliva represents fear or nervousness.

Recommended Affirmations: 7, 9, 16, 22, 25 and 31
Reiki Positions: A1, C1, C3 and C6 for ten minutes each, plus the elbows and the mouth.
Dietary and Other Suggestions:

- Apply pressure to the center of the line between the upper teeth and gums, and rotatory pressure at the sides of the elbows.

- Use glycerine mouthwash.

THE NOSE

Your nose represents your ego.

Colds

Colds are attempts to give you rest from the conflicts and discomforts in your life. They point out that you need to look at your conflicts in silence. If you respect the cold's purpose, it will leave you cleansed and stronger than before. Colds also result from unacknowledged feelings of hurt, loneliness, disapproval, rejection, guilt, fear, envy, sadness, disappointment and so on. When our ego fails to realize our potential, we get a stuffy nose; when it cries, we get a runny nose. Sometimes colds also stem from a fear of having to return to a situation you dislike or dread. Finally, colds sometimes occur simply because one resigns oneself to expecting them.

Recommended Affirmations: 7, 16 and 22–25

Reiki Positions: A1 (on the sides of the nose), A2–A3, A5–A6, B1–B4, B7, C3, C6, D1–D2 and the sides of the ribcage.

Dietary and Other Suggestions:

To overcome a cold and prevent recurring colds:

- Take two tablespoons of wheat-grass juice thrice a day.
- Drink carrot and spinach juice mixed in a 5:2 ratio thrice a day.
- Drink plenty of fluids generally.
- Heat some powdered black pepper and basil leaves in a glass of water and mix in two teaspoons of honey and one teaspoon each of ginger juice and lemon juice. Drink this thrice each day, including once just before bed.
- Thrice a day, pour two drops of cinnamon oil into hot water and breathe in the vapours for ten minutes; then rub a few drops of cinnamon oil on your temples, sinuses and chest. Pour a few drops of cinnamon oil into your warm bathwater.
- Eat some finely grated apple with honey and lemon juice every day.

- Eat fresh grapes every morning.
- Take chopped garlic twice or thrice a day.
- Cut down on dairy products, meats, eggs, starch and sugar.
- If the cold is accompanied by fever, eat plenty of raw fruits, especially citrus fruits, and vegetables including onions and garlic for two to three days.
- Keep yourself warm, but only to the extent that your body does not need to spend energy. Do not wear extra clothes, cover yourself with too many blankets or overheat the room.
- Stop smoking.
- Go for a one-mile walk, if you have the energy.
- Take leave from work for a day or two.
- Visualize an army of microscopic scavengers cleaning up germs with a powerful disinfectant spray, or imagine breathing in a healing, milky-white light and exhaling reddish-brown vapours carrying all the rubbish out of your body.

Nosebleeds

Nosebleeds come from the blood vessels just inside the nose at the septum, which divides the nose in two. Nosebleeds can be caused by colds, hypertension, a blood disorder, injury, excessive sneezing or sinus problems. On the metaphysical level it shows a desperate, unfulfilled need to be noticed, recognized and approved by others.

Recommended Affirmations: 21, 26–27 and 31

Reiki Positions: A1 (but on the sides of the nose, between the forehead and lips), A4–A6, B6 and D1 (across the shoulder blades) and D2. Then place one hand on the bleeding nostril and the other at the back of A4.

Dietary and Other Suggestions:

- Give your nose one good, vigorous blow to clear out any clots.
- Plug the bleeding side with a sterile cotton ball dipped in white vinegar and pinch the softer part of the nose for five to seven minutes. Repeat if necessary.
- Use ice-cold compresses at the bridge of the nose.

- Sit upright in a chair, tilt the head forward, and pinch the nostrils. Breathe through your mouth. Swallow or spit out any blood that goes to the back of the nose. Repeat after another fifteen minutes if necessary.
- Place two drops of lemon or onion juice into the nostrils.
- To prevent nosebleeds if you tend to get them, take two bananas with a glass of milk sweetened with jaggery powder for two weeks, or eat coconut first thing in the morning for a week.
- Stop smoking.

Sinus Problems

Sinuses are spaces in the facial bones, lined with mucous membranes through which mucous normally travels to the nose. During a cold, however, these ducts get congested and mucous accumulates, often causing inflammation that results in sinusitis. Hay fever, allergies and pollution can also cause sinusitis. The patient feels pain in the forehead and cheeks, especially when stooping forward or coughing. The sense of smell grows weak.

Metaphysically speaking, sinus problems can indicate that you feel uncomfortable, challenged or just irritated by someone who lives with you and is part of your life. Take rest and try to regain your freedom and strength.

Recommended Affirmations: 5, 16 and 22
Reiki Positions: A1 for 10 minutes and A2, A5, B1, D1 and D2 for five minutes each, twice a day.
Dietary and Other Suggestions:

- Step up your intake of garlic, horseradish or Cajun spice, ginger, cinnamon, mustard, fresh fruits and vegetables, hot soups, herbal tea and fruit and vegetable juices.
- Use an ionizer while working on a computer and, especially, in your bedroom at night.
- Inhale a drop or two of eucalyptus oil and lemon juice from a paper handkerchief.
- Reduce your intake of dairy products.
- Do *jal neti* (the nasal douche) using a teaspoon of table salt and a pinch of baking soda in two cups of lukewarm water.

Learn the technique from a yoga teacher if possible, or from a good book.

- Apply cold packs to the nape of the neck and the bridge of the nose.
- Rinse the inside of your nose with salt water, in a mixture of one tablespoon salt to one quart of water.
- Using your thumb and index finger, apply and release pressure on:
  - the tips of the smaller toes.
  - just below the tip of the big-toe nail.
  - the junction of the foot and the middle toe.
  - the arch of the foot, in line with the gap between the first and second toes.

Teeth and Gums

The teeth represent our ability to analyze facts and express our truth to others without any fears of their disapproval. Dental problems can also mirror prolonged inner disharmony involving the first and third chakras. Root-canal trouble indicates uprooting of our core beliefs, resulting in weakened self-confidence and decision-making ability.

The gums represent our ability to make decisions and to trust in life and in ourselves. When we develop self-esteem and start trusting life and ourselves, we stop hankering after others' love and approval. Bleeding gums show a distrust and lack of joy in our decisions. Pyorrhea shows our anger at not being able to make decisions.

Recommended Affirmations: 7, 9–10, 23, 26–27, 29–30 and 32–33

Reiki Positions: Provide Reiki to the affected teeth for ten minutes thrice a day, and to:

- A7 and D2 together (ten minutes).
- C3 and C6 (ten minutes).
- D7 and perineum (ten minutes).
- Big toes plus A3, A1, D5 and D7 for incisors.
- Second toe plus A1, B3, C1 and the hips for canines.
- Middle toe for premolars.

- Fourth toe for molars.
- Small toes for wisdom teeth.
- For pyorrhea, provide full-body Reiki daily for ten days, with an extra half hour at the mouth and an extra ten minutes at B5.

Dietary and Other Suggestions:

- Make a thick paste with five crushed cloves, ¼ teaspoon onion juice, ¼ teaspoon lemon juice, one teaspoon honey, an appropriate quantity of rock salt, any type of grain, ¼ teaspoon mustard oil and ¼ teaspoon turmeric powder. Immerse a small piece of ginger in this paste and hold it on the affected tooth.
- For toothaches, do not use hot compresses, even if they seem to bring relief. They may spread infection to the outer jaw.
- Use ice packs for fifteen minutes thrice a day on the aching cheek and at the joint between the thumb and index finger.
- Massage your gums by holding them between the thumb and index finger (with the latter on the outside).
- Rinse your mouth with salt water (do not swallow).
- Mix a pinch of salt in a tablespoon of baking soda and brush your teeth with it to remove plaque and tartar. Apply it along the gumlines with your finger. Rinse.
- To exercise the gums, follow your last meal of the day with sugarless chewing gum or cheese (the smellier the better).
- Eat at least one raw vegetable every day.
- Avoid sticky foods such as cake and pudding, and increase your intake of low-fat milk, yogurt, cheese, fresh fruits (especially citrus fruits) and vegetables.
- Stop smoking and cut down on alcohol, tea, sweet drinks and snacks between meals.

THE SCALP

Baldness

Apart from genetic influence, hair loss can also be due to pregnancy, anaemia, circulatory problems and thyroid disorders. Your scalp holds the roots of your hair, and when it gets tight and rigid it fails to provide the required breathing space. The hair then falls out and is, alas, not replaced. Relaxing the scalp with a mental suggestion or massage can delay the balding process.

The stress that stiffens the scalp results mainly from misalignment with your life purpose. Consider what you want to do, rather than what others want you to do. Look for professional work that satisfies you emotionally. Being misaligned with your life purpose may keep you in a state of perennial conflict, leading to a general distrust in life and a tendency to worry ceaselessly about things beyond your control. The world is perfect the way it is, and it needs to be accepted. It does not need you to control it.

Recommended Affirmations: 1, 5, 10, 16–17 and 22–24

Reiki Positions: To retard hair loss, provide Reiki at the affected areas for at least half an hour daily, and at A1 (at the sides of the nose and lips), B2, B7, C2, C5, D5, D7 and beneath the coccyx to the perineum for ten minutes each.

Dietary and Other Suggestions:

- Switch to a vegetarian diet.
- Take vitamins A, B complex, C and E under a physician's guidance.
- Take one tablespoon of wheat-grass juice thrice a day.
- Take one tablespoon of honey every day.
- Eat more legumes, peas, yogurt, yeast extracts, sweet potatoes, dried apricots, pumpkin seeds (especially for dry, dandruff-prone hair), and whole-wheat flour.
- Drink the juices of cabbage, ginger, alfalfa, asparagus, carrots, broccoli, green peppers and all leafy green vegetables.
- Massage your scalp with a mixture of lemon and garlic juice, applied with an onion cut in half. Leave it for ten minutes or so before bathing. Alternately, massage your scalp with warm almond oil, leave it for an hour and then wash it with a mild shampoo.

Psoriasis

Psoriasis is the accumulation of itchy, silvery scales on the buttocks and scalp, the soles of the feet and the backs of the wrists, elbows, knees and ankles. The toenails and fingernails may also lose their shine and develop ridges and pits as a result of abnormally faster skin-cell division. Psoriasis can result from stress, infection and some drugs. Metaphysically it represents a paradox—you want to be loved, but you fear closeness and other such emotions. Since you are not opening yourself up to receive love, your body is doing it for you—your scalp is being opened up with cracks and sores. Do not be afraid of being hurt, cheated, deceived or vulnerable; open yourself up to receive *and* to express love.

Recommended Affirmations: 14, 19, 21 and 28

Reiki Positions: Full-body Reiki with extra time on A2–A5 and affected areas.

Dietary and Other Suggestions:

- Eat more raw foods—more than half of every meal— especially ginger, papayas, pineapples, beetroots, carrots, spinach, and oranges.
- Do not leave your skin dry. Use body oil or jelly soon after your bath.
- Apply ice to the affected areas.
- Expose the affected area to sunlight for one hour each day. Use a sunscreen on the unaffected areas.
- Give up alcohol.
- Lose any excess weight.
- Do yoga nidra to a guided progressive-relaxation tape.

THE NECK

Neck pain can often be tracked down to a social interaction that caused you irritation, hurt, resentment or any other ill feeling. The stress of having faced, or having to face, an unpleasant situation tenses up the neck muscles so they can better absorb the shock. Stress that comes from anger, frustration or a desire to take revenge affects the jaws in particular. Prolonged stress in the neck may squeeze the nerves coming from the spinal cord and may necessitate surgery.

Stiff Neck

The neck carries the head above the body. Its flexibility represents that of our thoughts. If it is flexible, like the trunk of a healthy tree, it can weather many a storm. Rigid ways of thinking and behaving can invite problems: a stiff-necked attitude manifests itself as a stiff neck in order to draw your attention towards the need to soften your narrow, self-centered attitude. Be more flexible and tolerant; consider the opinions of others.

Recommended Affirmations: 4, 6, 30 and 35

Reiki Positions: A7 (but with both hands at the back on both sides of the neck), B2, B6–B7, C3 and C6, and the exact spot of stiffness or pain.

Natural/Dietary Supplements:

- Adopt a strictly vegetarian diet.
- Give up alcohol.
- Take plenty of the following vitamins from their natural sources: vitamin C (gooseberries, citrus fruits), vitamin B complex, (potatoes, preferably with skin; green vegetables; blueberries; pulses; seeds; beans; brown rice; brown bread; and betel nuts) and vitamin E (safflower oil, olive oil, nuts and avocados).
- Relieve stress through yoga nidra, pranayama and meditation.
- Do shankh prakshalan—a yogic kriya that cleans the digestive tract—under the guidance of an expert.
- Protect your neck from cold weather by using a neck wrap or muffler.
- Alternate the use of an ice pack and heating pad at the affected spot.
- Get yourself a vertical book holder so you don't have to bend your neck for long durations.
- Always use a straight-backed chair, and insert a rolled towel behind the small of your back.
- Do not sleep on your stomach. Sleep on your back, using a cervical pillow under the nape of the neck and an ordinary pillow under your knees *rather* than under your head.

Alternately, if you prefer to sleep on your side, choose the left side (aids in digestion) and bend your knees slightly towards your chest. Use a pillow or two to ensure that your head is horizontal. Thin, bony people can insert a small pillow between their knees as well.

- To lift objects from the ground: squat down, grasp the object and stand up by straightening your knees, keeping your spine erect.

Do the following exercises regularly:

- Rotate your shoulders clockwise and then anti-clockwise, twelve times each. Breathe in as you go up, out as you go down.

- Fold your arms at the elbows so that your fingers touch the neck-shoulder joint. Now bring your elbows forward and as close to each other as possible, and move them in a circle clockwise and then anti-clockwise twelve times each. Breathe in as you go up, out as you go down.

- Place your hands on your waist and try to join your elbows behind you. Bring them back to your sides and repeat twelve times. Breathe in as you bring your elbows back, out as you bring them forwards.

- Bend your neck forward and slowly rotate it in a large horizontal circle around an imaginary vertical axis through the centre of your neck. Go clockwise first, then anti-clockwise, twelve times each. Take care that the body below the neck, including the shoulders, stays still. Breathe in as you bring the neck back, out as you bring it forward.

- Breathe in and bend your neck sideways, first to the left. While breathing out, bring it slowly back to the centre and, without stopping, over towards the right shoulder. Breathe in, move your neck towards the left shoulder again and repeat twelve times.

- Slowly bend your neck about its vertical axis towards the left and then towards the right, going as far as you can go. Breathe in as you go left, out as you go right.

- Slowly bend your neck forwards. Bring it back and then, without stopping, bend it backwards as far as it will go.

Breathe in as you bring your neck back, out as you bring it forwards. Repeat twelve times.

- Cross your hands above your head. Slowly and simultaneously make a clockwise circle with your right arm and an anti-clockwise circle with your left arm. Breathe in as you go up, out as you go down. Repeat twelve times. Now reverse the direction of each arm and repeat twelve more times.
- Repeat the above exercise with arms rotating at your sides rather than in front of you.
- Spread your arms horizontally, with your palms facing forwards. Slowly start bending your palms backwards, as far as they will go. Hold your breath and stay there for a count of two, then bring them back to the original position. Breathe in as you bring your hands back, out as you bring them forwards. Repeat twelve times.
- Lie on your back with your head overhanging the edge of the bed. Let your head relax by dropping it back as far as it can comfortably go, then slowly raising it. Hold for five deep, slow breaths and then let the head go slowly down again. Repeat five times every morning or evening.

THE THROAT

The throat chakra represents our creativity and our ability to take a stand (about anything, but especially our own needs) and keep our lives in order. Some people find it difficult to swallow a particular comment or situation but equally difficult to convey their real feelings, needs, desires and wants lest they hurt someone or tarnish their own image. Those who find it difficult to stand up for themselves are prone to throat problems, as are those whose creativity is somehow stifled—professionally or otherwise.

The throat chakra is where we process changes in our lives. Resistance to change makes us cough—so whenever someone coughs, it shows the need to examine the change he or she is confronting and his or her willingness to live with that change.

Hyper- / Hypo-thyroidism

Hyperthyroidism is the condition of a hyperactive thyroid gland, resulting in heightened heart rate and metabolism and general nervousness. Because the body consumes vital nutrients and burns calories at an accelerated pace, the patient may lose weight (in spite of a good appetite; in fact, appetite may increase) and experience fatigue, irritability, goiter, sweating, sensitivity to heat and bulging eyes. Hyperthyroidism can result from excessive iodine intake. Antibodies developed in the thyroid tend to stimulate this gland to overactivity.

Hypothyroidism occurs when the body develops antibodies against its own thyroid gland, resulting in reduced hormone production. Symptoms include fatigue, drowsiness, apathy, goitre, forgetfulness, weight gain, muscle weakness, sensitivity to cold, constipation and dry skin and hair. The body loses the ability to convert beta carotene into vitamin A, resulting in a build-up of beta carotene in the blood and tissues, which in turn give the skin a yellowish tinge. The hands may also show a tendency to tremble when outstretched; this stems from extreme anger at the sense that one has been ignored rather than favoured for some responsibility, attention or favour.

Recommended Affirmations: 5, 16, 18, 22, 26–27 and 30

Reiki Positions (for both thyroid problems): A1, A6–A7, B1, across the shoulder blades, C3, C6 and D5.

Dietary and Other Suggestions:

- For either thyroid problem, boil five spoonfuls of dry coriander seeds in a glass of water, filter it and drink it twice a day.
- For hyperthyroidism, adopt a diet rich in protein, whole grains, potatoes and dairy products. Give up coffee, tea, cola, chocolate, alcohol and smoking.
- For hyperthyroidism, place more of the colour green in your surroundings, wear green more often and meditate on green for ten minutes daily. For hypothyroidism, do the same with blue.

Laryngitis

Laryngitis is the inflammation of the voice box (larynx), resulting in hoarseness or loss of voice. It can be acute and short-lived, or it can be chronic. Laryngitis shows such extreme anger, hopelessness and disgust with the authorities or seniors in one's life that one finds it futile even to speak of it.

Recommended Affirmations: 31
Reiki Positions: A6–A7, B4, C3, C6 and D1.
Dietary and Other Suggestions:

- Drink plenty of fluids, though not coffee, tea, cola, orange juice, milk or anything cold.
- Inhale steam vapours for ten minutes thrice a day.
- Apply and release pressure on the web between the thumb and index finger (more towards the finger side) and at the bottom outer corner of the thumbnail.
- Gargle with a mixture of red sage and fresh lemon juice.
- Rest your voice completely. Do not even whisper.
- Have you neck, back muscles and upper chest massaged.
- Apply a cold compress to the back of the neck, near the bottom of the skull.

Quinsy

Quinsy is a severe inflammation of the tonsils, throat or adjacent parts, accompanied by fever. It stems from a deep-seated belief that one simply cannot speak up for oneself and ask for one's needs. The pain may also involve the ear, resulting in difficulty swallowing and speaking.

Recommended Affirmations: 6 and 31
Reiki Positions: A6–A7
Dietary and Other Suggestions:

- Drink more fluids, especially fresh fruit juices.
- Gargle with red sage.
- Apply a cold compress around the neck.

Sore Throat

Inflammation of any kind is usually the result of suppressed anger and/or fear. A sore throat occurs when we swallow instead of expressing our feelings. Normally, the mucous-coated pharynx (at the back of the throat) traps most of the germs that enter our body through inhalation, and saves us from infection. Every day, a quart of mucous goes down to our stomach, where the germs trapped in it are killed with hydrochloric acid. The remaining germs are killed by the army of cells devoted to this purpose. However, when we feel unloved, sad, disappointed or hurt by someone's unfriendly remark, the body tries instinctively to repeat what it learnt in infancy: at a deep subconscious level the throat begins subtly to mimic the movements associated with sucking at the mother's breast. As this is a futile exercise, the movements tire the pharynx and cause the mucous to dry up, leaving the pharynx exposed to invading germs. The germs then have a field day, and we feel the results in our sinuses, nostrils and, of course, throat.

To prevent sore throats, take stock of your unpleasant feelings from time to time. And whenever you feel uneasy, ask yourself exactly why.

Recommended Affirmations: 10, 17
Reiki Positions: A2, A4, A6–A7, B4, C3, C6
Dietary and Other Suggestions:

- Switch to a diet rich in fruits and vegetables, especially carrots, spinach, avocados and olive oil.
- Gargle with hot lemon water stirred with half a teaspoon of salt.
- Take plenty of fluids, except coffee, tea, cola, orange juice and milk.
- Give up alcohol and smoking.
- Inhale steam thrice a day.
- Stir one tablespoon of horseradish and one teaspoon of ground cloves into a glass of warm water. Keep stirring as you sip it slowly.
- Raise the head end of your bed four to six inches to prevent stomach acids from moving up to your throat.
- Change your toothbrush every month, especially when you feel that you are about to fall sick. Change it again when you have recovered fully.

Tonsillitis

Inflammation of the tonsils—the two masses of tissue at the back of the throat—is more common in children than adults. Metaphysically it indicates fear, bottled-up emotion, unexpressed creativity or a deep conflict that has been suppressed.

Recommended Affirmations: 9, 16

Reiki Positions: A1, A3, A5–A7, B1 (T variation), B5, and D5, with an extra ten minutes under the lower jaw.

Dietary and Other Suggestions:

- Cut out milk.
- Cut out biscuits, cakes and table sugar. De-stress yourself with progressive relaxation or meditation.
- Drink more fluids, especially citrus juices.
- Gargle with a mixture of red sage and fresh lemon juice.
- Drink ¼ teaspoon garlic juice thrice a day.
- Apply a cold compress around the neck.
- Inhale salt water. The water should be as salty as a tear.
- Those who know how to perform *jal neti kriya* may do that as well.

THE RESPIRATORY SYSTEM

Breathing comprises two motions: inhaling (taking in new thoughts and ideas that are most relevant to your life right now) and exhaling (letting go of stale thoughts and ideas). Breathing also represents freedom and the ability to come in contact with our unknown or lesser feelings and emotions. The fear of being in touch with things we don't want to feel or confront (the painful knots of past experiences, present in our aural body as blocks) keeps us from breathing fully. Respiratory problems, therefore, indicate problems in these areas: inhalation, exhalation, freedom and willingness to confront our blocks. If and when you are afflicted with a respiratory problem, ask yourself: What is it that you don't want to share with others? What is it that you don't want to take from others? What makes you feel that your freedom is inhibited? What is it that you want to control in your life? What keeps you from fulfilling your dreams? Metaphysically speaking, if you want something more in your life, focus not on receiving but on giving—receiving will take care of itself, just as a focus on improving your exhalation results automatically in rich inhalation as well. Authorities on breathing reveal that in order to exhale more completely, we must learn to let go of all that is unnecessary in our lives: the kind of work we do, the material things we hardly use, the personal ambitions that are not really ours but were imposed on us by others.

Asthma

Asthma can result from allergies or infection. Asthmatic attacks, during which breathing grows difficult and is accompanied by a wheezing sound, occur when inflammation or a muscular spasm causes the bronchial passages to contract. Attacks can last anywhere from a few minutes to a few hours; prolonged attacks should be referred to a medical professional. Asthma usually develops in childhood; in adults it can develop as a result of recurrent chest infections or heart ailments.

At some level, asthmatic people feel a lack of space for themselves in their lives, or think they do not deserve to live for themselves. Housewives, eldest sons and others who have self-abnegating roles that involve 'living for others' are particularly prone. Asthma is your body's expression of deep-seated feelings of being unloved, deserted, abandoned and devoid of emotional support. People who eternally yearn for others' love do so for three reasons—they become too dependent on others' love, they do good works for others mainly because they feel they 'have to', and they carry a deep-rooted belief that they are not worthy of others' love, and must thus make an extraordinary display of their love for others in order to get some back. The right attitude towards receiving anything external is to wish for it and do what you can to bring it about, but also to avoid letting your happiness depend it.

Recommended Affirmations: 7
Reiki Positions:
- During an attack, B1, B2 and B4 for ten minutes or more.

- Between attacks, A1, A3–A5, B2, B5, B7, D1 and D5.
- Provide Reiki for half an hour for twenty-one consecutive days to both sides of the torso (one after the other), a hand's breadth below the armpits, and to the chest with both hands. Keep your thumbs tucked within your palm.

Dietary and Other Suggestions:

- Eat radishes with honey.
- Cut down on table salt.
- Reduce your intake of dairy products, eggs, nuts and dried fruits (especially peanuts), apricots, fish and seafood.
- Increase your intake of fresh fruits and vegetables such as garlic, onions, leafy green vegetables, bananas, grapefruit, watercress, pulses, dried figs, sunflower seeds, carrots and spinach.
- Increase your intake of potatoes, brown rice, soybeans, whole-grain cereals and bread, and natural sources of vitamin B6 such as yeast extracts, wheat germ and oats.
- Boil chopped turnips in a little water and take a few teaspoons of this syrup thrice a day.
- Cut out white sugar and white flour, and all foods containing colouring agents and other additives—especially MBSB (metabisulfite benzoates) and MSG (monosodium glutamate).
- Run your air-conditioner on the maximum or 're-circulate' setting.
- Prop the head side of your bed four to six inches to prevent stomach acid from moving into your throat.
- Avoid going out in very cold weather. If you must, wear a scarf over your nose and mouth.
- Cut out smoking and alcohol.
- Do some deep, slow, relaxed breathing every morning.
- Keep an ionizer switched on in the bedroom.
- Do yogasanas in the corpse posture, shoulder stand, cobra, back-roll and fish positions.
- Do past-life regression therapy.

Bronchitis

Bronchitis is an inflammation of the large passages (bronchi) that carry air through the windpipe to the lungs. You are more prone to bronchitis when the conflicts in your life become acute, when anger sets in or when an unexpected, unpleasant change confronts you—in short, when life hands you something you'd rather cough out.

Recommended Affirmations: 7, 16 and 22–25
Reiki Positions: A1–A7, B1–B2, B5, C3, C6, D1, D5 and D7.
Dietary and Other Suggestions:

- Reduce your intake of dairy products, eggs, nuts, fish and seafood.
- Stop smoking. Protect yourself from passive smoke. If you absolutely cannot quit, drink a glass of milk every day
- Drink lots of fluids, minus tea, coffee, cola and alcohol.
- Eat a garlic clove thrice a day.
- Eat more fresh fruits and vegetables, and drink their juices and soups.
- Cut out white sugar and white flour, yeast and all foods containing colouring agents and other additives—especially MBSB (metabisulfite benzoates) and MSG (monosodium glutamate).
- Boil chopped turnips in a little water and take a few teaspoons of this syrup thrice a day.
- Avoid dry, over-heated rooms and sudden changes in temperature.
- Massage the soles of your feet with mustard oil before going to bed.
- Instead of using expectorants, inhale steam vapours from a bowl.

Emphysema

Emphysema is a condition wherein tiny air sacs in the lungs get enlarged due to inflammation, swelling and excessive mucous production, a disorder marked by air-filled expansion of body tissues and abnormal enlargement of the air sacs in the lungs causing breathlessness The patient finds it difficult to breathe and is often beset by persistent, painful coughing fits, which put extra strain on the heart. The patient also tires very easily. Emphysema represents grief, depression or an inability to accept life as a gift or live it to its fullest. It stems from an excessive desire for the love, affection and approval that were not adequately provided during childhood.

Most emphysema patients are smokers. Smoking is a way of filling ourselves up with smoke as a substitute to love, which also gives us a façade of being self-sufficient. It also represents their belief that they are unworthy of the joy of life. Instead of letting smoking deny you the joy of life, recognize your abnormal hunger for love and affection without feeling guilty about it. As a first step, write down this acknowledgement and share it with yourself or even with some close, understanding friends. This will take a load off your lungs.

Recommended Affirmations: 16, 26–27 and 31

Reiki Positions: Full-body treatment with extra time on A6, B1–B2, B4, C3, C6 and D1–D2 every day for at least a month.

Dietary and Other Suggestions:

- Eat fruits and vegetables rich in vitamin C (citrus fruits, gooseberries, black currants), beta carotene (carrots, apricots, spinach, mangoes, papayas), and vitamin E (whole-grain cereals, sunflower seeds).
- Drink lots of wheat-grass juice.
- Avoid dairy products.
- Stop smoking. Protect yourself from passive smoke.
- Wear loose clothes. Train yourself to breathe slowly, smoothly, deeply and correctly using your abdomen, your chest and your shoulders.
- Do some regular exercise such as swimming, Sudarshan Kriya, tai chi or Surya Namaskar (but at a slower pace and with fewer cycles).
- Keep an ionizer switched on in the bedroom.

Pneumonia/Tuberculosis

Pneumonia and tuberculosis represent a tiring conflict between your ego and the way your life is unfolding. Pneumonia, marked by chest pain, fever, coughing and difficult breathing, is an inflammation of one or both lungs, occurring when the alveoli (air sacs) fill with fluid and white blood cells. Pneumonia can be caused by bacteria, a virus, fungi or other micro-organisms, and is most likely to occur when the immune system is weak.

Tuberculosis is a contagious bacterial infection involving the formation of nodules called tubercles in various tissues, especially the lungs. Symptoms include fatigue, coughing, difficulty breathing, blood in the sputum, loss of appetite (and weight) and fever, but they often remain dormant until the body is weakened by some other disease. Tuberculosis occurs when one allows oneself to be possessed by selfish, cruel, vengeful thoughts.

Recommended Affirmations: 4–5, 7–9, 12, 16, 22, 24

Reiki Treatment: Physicians must attend to both these diseases; Reiki should be used only as a supportive aid. In non-crisis situations, apply Reiki daily so long as the fever remains (usually three to four days). If the fever lingers, continue group Reiki with symbols until it breaks. During Reiki treatment, have the patient lie on his or her back with the head and upper chest slightly elevated. You may have to slip your hands under the patient's body for D positions.

Reiki Positions: A1–A7, B1–B2, B5, C3, C6, B1 and D1 together, D2, D5 and D7 plus the wrists, base of the thumb and top of the shoulders.

Dietary and Other Suggestions:

For tuberculosis:

- Eat more grains, pulses, fresh fruits, vegetables and foods rich in vitamin D and vitamin B12, such as eggs, oily fish and dairy products.
- Drink a glass a day of pineapple, unripe banana and orange juice, the latter stirred with a pinch of salt and two teaspoons of honey.
- Avoid exertion. Get plenty of rest.

For pneumonia:

- For a few days, eat only fresh fruits and vegetables and their juices, especially wheat-grass juice. Gradually introduce

whole grains and proteins under the guidance of a
professional naturopath.

- Stop smoking. Protect yourself from passive smoke.
- Avoid dairy products.
- Eat lots of dark-green leafy vegetables, especially spinach
  and kale.
- Eat fruits and vegetables rich in vitamin C (citrus fruits,
  gooseberries, black currants) and beta carotene (carrots,
  apricots, spinach, mangoes, papayas) and vitamin E (whole-
  grain cereals, sunflower seeds).
- Drink lots of fluids, especially fruit juices and vegetable
  soups, in small quantities throughout the day. Avoid coffee,
  tea, and cola.
- Do Surya Namaskar, but at a slower pace with fewer cycles.
- Keep an ionizer switched on in the bedroom.

THE BREASTS

The breasts represent femininity. Problems relating to the breasts
may indicate the woman's rejection of her own femininity or a
feeling that she has been rejected by others. Lumps, cysts and
actual breast cancer indicate sorrow or dissatisfaction with a
lack of attention from one's life partner. Such problems are
particularly likely in women whose partners have died or left
them for someone else, women whose partners for some reason
lose interest in their breasts during foreplay, and women who
delay child-bearing or never have children at all. Apart from
getting breasts their due attention, the key to healthy breasts is
to express either to oneself or to one's partner the hurt of being
deprived of this attention. Because breasts also represent
motherhood, breast problems can indicate attempts to
overprotect a person or an aspect of one's life, or a tendency to
consider others more important than oneself.

Recommended Affirmations: 11, 14, 16, 27–28 and 32
Reiki Positions:

- Cover both breasts with your cupped palms and channel
  Reiki for twenty to twenty-five minutes. If the patient is

someone else, keep your palms an inch or two above the chest.
- B4, B7 (for at least twenty minutes) and D5.

Dietary and Other Suggestions:

Stick to a vegetarian diet low in fat and high in fibre: whole grains, fresh fruits and vegetables, and soybean products. Eat foods rich in magnesium (whole-grain cereals, dried figs, nuts, pulses, garlic, wheat-grass juice, parsley and leafy green vegetables), calcium (milk, cheese and dark-green leafy vegetables), vitamin B complex (potatoes, preferably with skin, pulses, green vegetables, seeds, beans, brown rice, blueberries, betel nuts, brown bread) and vitamin C (citrus fruits, gooseberries).

- Cut down on salty foods, animal fats, tea, coffee, cola and chocolate.
- Cut out smoking and alcohol.
- Do regular yogasanas (especially bow and cobra) and Surya Namaskar
- Do deep-breathing exercises.
- Alternate hot and cold packs on the breasts.
- Lose any excess weight.
- Examine your breasts regularly to check that (a) the nipples move when you raise and lower your arms; (b) there is no discharge from the nipples when they are squeezed gently; (c) there is no flaky skin or rash on the nipples; (d) there are no lumps anywhere on either breast.

THE SHOULDERS

The shoulders represent our ability to identify and accept our responsibilities wisely, and shoulder them joyously. Often we yearn to shoulder an esteemed responsibility but doubt if it will ever be granted, so we hide it from conscious thought. Shoulder pain manifests this desire. Alternately, burdens we have been carrying or feel we *should* be carrying can manifest themselves as shoulder pain.

So become aware of what is causing pain in your shoulders.

Admit consciously what you want to achieve or acquire; learn to delegate responsibilities; and do not be afraid to take on the responsibilities that are really your own. Shoulder them joyously. It is actually the Latent Oneness that will take on your load, if only you show your willingness and commitment. Often what becomes tiring is not the responsibility but the unwillingness and resistance to shoulder it. Responsibility is 'response' + 'ability'. Once you make a decision to take responsibility, the ability to do so comes on its own.

Recommended Affirmations: 1, 5, 7, 9, 14, 16, 18–19 and 22

Reiki Positions:

- D1–D3, biceps, elbows and wrists.

Dietary and Other Suggestions:

- Eat plenty of fresh fruits, vegetables and other foods rich in vitamin A (mangoes, cantaloupe, melon), selenium (whole-grain cereals), and vitamin E (avocados, nuts, sunflower seeds).
- Drink carrot, parsley, ginger and broccoli juices.
- Avoid citrus fruits, tomatoes, potatoes, peppers (other than black), eggplant, white flour, all sweets and processed foods.
- Avoid smoking and alcohol.
- Train yourself to sit, stand, walk and sleep with correct posture (see 'The Back', below)
- Get regular massages.
- Do the exercises recommended for stiff neck (above).
- Lose any excess weight.

THE BACK

The back is a metaphor for support and moral uprightness. Back problems indicate a perceived lack of support. While the upper and lower back relate to emotional and material support, the middle of the back relates to guilt. Upper-back problems afflict those who hold back their love and affection for others, or have suffered an emotional setback, or feel envious of people they love. Lower-back pain results from responsibilities (real or imagined) that make one feel torn yet unable to delegate. If you have back pain, trust others and open yourself up to the universe that created you. When you love and trust others, you get love and trust in return.

Recommended Affirmations: 1, 3, 5, 9, 16, 22, 24 and 30

Reiki Positions: In addition to A1, C1, C3 and C6, provide Reiki for ten minutes each at:

- D1–D3 for upper-back pain
- D3–D4 for middle-back pain
- D5–D7 for lower-back pain

For chronic pain, provide Reiki along the length of the spine, shifting down one hand's breadth every five or ten minutes.

Dietary and Other Suggestions:

- Eat plenty of cabbage, guavas and papayas.
- Cut down on coffee, tea, chocolate and cola.
- Lose any excess weight, especially by cutting down on fat and sugar.
- Alternate hot and cold packs every half hour.

Posture Care:

- If you must lift a heavy object from the floor, squat down on your haunches, grasp the object and then stand up, keeping your spine erect. When you carry a heavy object, try to hold equal weight in each of your hands.
- To get out of bed in the morning, turn on to your side, slide to the edge of the bed and then roll up and out of bed, letting your legs come off the bedside first.
- When seated, keep your spine erect—do not allow a gap between the back of the chair and the lumbar curve of your spine. Keep your buttocks as close to the back of the chair as possible.
- When brushing your teeth at the wash basin, bend your knees to keep your spine erect.
- Sleep on your left side, keeping your head horizontal by supporting it with pillows. Keep a pillow between your knees. Alternately, sleep on your back with a rolled towel under the nape of your neck and a pillow under your knees.

Exercises:

- *Exercise 1*

— Lie down on your back with arms at your sides and your

head to one side. Take ten slow, deep breaths and relax for
five minutes.
— Keeping your palms and forearms on the floor, lift yourself
until your elbows are right under your shoulders. Take ten
slow, deep breaths and relax for five minutes, letting your
lower back relax completely.
— Start straightening your arms, slowly pushing up the upper
half of your chest in the process. Hold this position for a
count of ten and go back to step two. Repeat ten times,
trying to reach a little higher each time.

■ *Exercise 2*
— Stand upright with your feet slightly apart. Place your hands
at the back of your waist.
— Bend your trunk as far backwards as you can without bending
your knees or losing your balance. Come back to the original
position slowly. Repeat ten times.

■ *Exercise 3*
Lie down on your back. Close your eyes and imagine a white
cloud of healing light hovering over the area where you feel
pain. Imagine it descending on the pain, penetrating it and
quickly repairing all the painful cells to bring you relief.

■ *Exercise 4* (Bhujangasana)
Lie on your stomach. Keeping your pelvis on the floor, push
yourself up with your hands, raising your shoulders and slowly
arching your back. Take ten breaths and slowly return to the
original position. Repeat twice.

■ *Exercise 5*
Lie on your back with your feet on the floor and knees bent.
Cross your arms and keep your hands on your shoulders. Raise
your head and shoulders off the floor as high as you can while
keeping your back on floor. Hold for one second, then return
to the original position and repeat.

■ *Exercise 6*
Lie on your stomach and raise your left arm and right leg
simultaneously. Hold for one second, then repeat with the right
arm and left leg.

Spine Fractures / Slipped Discs

Spine fractures indicate a rigid, biased, perhaps arrogant attitude. To reduce your chances of a spine fracture, learn to flow with life.

Discs are the spine's shock absorbers. Healthy discs have a soft, pulpy centre with a fibrous outer casing. When the casing is damaged, the soft centre bulges out, and is then called a 'slipped disc'. Slipped discs often occur in the lower back, causing dull but severe pain, spasms and sometimes numbness in the leg or foot. It may be difficult to stand erect. Slipped discs show indecision and a feeling of being unsupported by life.

Recommended Affirmations: 5, 9–10, 16 and 22–25

Reiki Positions: B5–B6, C2–C7, D5 and the affected area for ten minutes each.

Dietary and Other Suggestions:

- Use a hot-water bottle or infra-red lamp on the affected spot.
- Sleep on a firm mattress.
- Follow the rules of right posture given in 'The Back', above. Do not resume your unhealthy postures once you are relieved of the problem. It may recur.

THE BLOOD

The blood represents energy and joy. The heart represents our capacity to feel and give due place in our lives to emotions such as love. Blood circulation represents our capacity to feel and express our feelings in positive ways. When we start focusing too much on what we think are important events, we lose our sensitivity to the small, day-to-day joys, and over time we stop expecting or experiencing joy. Under these conditions the heart, like an unwatered plant, can start to shrivel and wither, and may give us a stroke. Similarly, bleeding suggests that joy is running out of our lives, and blood clots show a freezing or entrapping of joy.

Anaemia/Arteriosclerosis

Haemoglobin is the pigmented red-blood cell that carries oxygen. When the haemoglobin count goes down, less oxygen reaches the tissues, resulting in fatigue and weakness or, in more serious cases, palpitations, breathlessness, swollen feet or general pain. This condition is known as anaemia. Anaemia can result from the simple inability to produce enough red blood cells, or from a genetic abnormality. Haemolytic anaemia is a condition in which red blood cells break down faster than they can be replaced.

An inability to absorb vitamin B12 may lead to pernicious anaemia. Iron-deficiency anaemia is caused by poor diet or loss of blood, as through heavy menstrual periods or internal bleeding from cancer or an ulcer. Megaloblastic anaemia arises from a shortage of folic acid, one of the B vitamins. Blood diseases such as leukaemia can also lead to anaemia.

Arteriosclerosis is caused by thickening and loss of elasticity in the artery walls. Symptoms can include chest pain, leg pain, and disturbances in vision, speech and use of the limbs.

Since blood represents joy and energy, the arteries are the carriers of joy. Circulation problems may indicate a lack of joy in one's life, or stagnant, perhaps negative ideas that lack the energy to flow freely. Anaemic people tend to lack joy, optimism, flexibility, confidence, dynamism and courage in their lives, and arteriosclerosis patients tend toward tension, rigidity and narrow-mindedness. These patients need to be more positive about life, more open to joy and love.

Recommended Affirmations: 8, 16, 21, 26 and 30
Reiki Positions: A4–A5, top of the head, B1, B3, B5, C2–C7 and full-body with mental healing.
Dietary and Other Suggestions:

- Eat plenty of leafy green vegetables, strawberries, parsley, horseradish, nettles, apricots, pumpkin seeds, walnuts, raisins, brewer's yeast, wheat germ and fortified breakfast cereals.
- Take dairy products in moderation. Replace them with soya milk and tofu.

- Mix carrot and spinach juice in a 2:1 ratio and drink it daily.
- Have a tomato salad or a glass of orange juice with every meal.
- Regular exercises such as yoga, Surya Namaskar and tai chi provide the best possible protection.

Angina Pectoris

Angina, caused by inadequate blood supply during strenuous work, is experienced as sudden immobilizing spasms in the upper chest, accompanied by exhaustion, nausea, a choking sensation, and a feeling of impending death. The spasms last for several minutes or more, and can spread to the left or both arms. Note that lying down during an attack may aggravate the discomfort.

When we cease to see ourselves as a part of the Latent Oneness, our spirit constricts, and the barriers within our being result in fears. These fears make us strive for power, and we squeeze our heart in the process. If you suffer from angina, wake up to your fears—accept them and go beyond them. Accept and give, without any inhibitions, all that expresses love and beauty.

Recommended Affirmations: 9 and 12
Reiki Positions: A1–A7, B1–B6 and D1–D2. For a nervous heart, channel Reiki to A2–A3, D1–D2 and D5 plus both sides of the chest, a hand's breath below the armpits.
Dietary and Other Suggestions:

- Seek professional medical help.
- Eat plenty of raw or lightly cooked vegetables, fresh fruits, salads, whole-grain cereals, oatmeal porridge and oat bran (to reduce cholesterol).
- Take a tablespoon of wheat-grass juice thrice a day.
- Replace animal and dairy products with soya milk and unsaturated margarine.
- Cut out white salt, white sugar, white flour, tea, coffee, cola, smoking and large amounts of alcohol.
- Avoid stress—take it easy.
- Do slow, deep-breathing exercises.

- Do yoga nidra meditation regularly.
- Raise the head end of your bed four to six inches.
- See 'Heart Attack', below, for more on cardiovascular health.

Atherosclerosis

Atherosclerosis is a nodular hardening of the arteries because of fatty deposits therein. When LDL (low-density cholesterol) accumulates in the blood, it eventually congeals to form fatty streaks on the artery wall. HDL (high-density cholesterol) retards this formation. Metaphysically, atherosclerosis indicates a blocking of the joy in life, and a fear of enjoyment.

Recommended Affirmations: 21
Reiki Positions: B1, B3, B5, C3 and C7 for at least five to seven minutes each.

Dietary and Other Suggestions:

- Eat plenty of citrus fruits, strawberries, avocados, tomatoes, carrots, spinach, potatoes, rice, soybeans, barley, spirulina, nuts, oatmeal porridge, oat bran and corn bran.
- Drink skimmed milk and cook with canola, peanut, olive, corn or safflower oil.
- Eat a clove of garlic with each meal.
- Continue with rice.
- Cut out meat, saturated fats, butter, cheese, hydrogenated oil, white salt, white sugar, white flour, tea, coffee, cola, eggs, smoking and alcohol.
- Drink a teaspoonful of Metamucil or any other psyllium-seed product in water thrice a day.
- Lose any excess weight.
- Do tai chi, Surya Namaskar (slowly), yoga, yoga nidra or any other progressive relaxation technique.

Heart Attack

A heart attack, or myocardial infarction, is a sudden decrease in the heart's ability to function. It occurs when the coronary artery gets blocked or damaged, cutting off the heart's blood supply. (A partial blockage may lead to angina pectoris; see above.) Among the early signs are uncomfortable pressure, a squeezing sensation, feeble pain in the centre of the chest (perhaps radiating into the shoulders, arms, neck or jaw), shortness of breath, fatigue, dizziness and nausea.

Heart attacks occur when long-suppressed aggressive energy, having no outlet, turns within and essentially 'explodes' the heart. Do not wait for big things to make you happy—the most precious things in one's life are small joys, for not only do they give meaning to life, but they also keep our heart from hardening along the way. Pay attention to your emotions and accept life as it comes, and your heart will keep its flexibility.

Recommended Affirmations: 8, 16, 21, 26 and 30. Work on forgiving all those you hold grudges against. Read a few quotations from the author's *Little Book of Forgiveness* (or any other book on forgiveness) every day.

Reiki Treatment:

- Seek urgent medical assistance. You can provide Reiki to the back of the heart with both hands (at B3, B5–B6, D1, D3 and D5) on the way to the hospital.
- To prevent heart attacks, provide Reiki to B1, C3, C6 and D3, plus B2–B3 and B5–B6 if you have time.

Dietary and Other Suggestions:

- In an emergency, hold the tips of the patient's little fingers and whirl them around. Give the patient five cloves of garlic immediately upon the onset of an attack. Once the emergency has passed, the patient should continue taking garlic cloves boiled in milk.
- Increase your intake of fresh fruits (especially citrus fruits, gooseberries and guavas), green vegetables, whole grains, onions (those at risk need to have a boiled onion every morning) and garlic.
- Give up smoking and alcohol. For middle-aged and older people, a daily glass or two of red wine (give Reiki to it before drinking to enhance its healing effect) can help, but opt for this *only* if you have the self-control to stop at this dose.
- Cut out mustard oil, hydrogenated oils and saturated margarines from your cooking regimen, and cut out animal fats, butter and cream. You can have oily fish (tuna, salmon,

sardines) twice a week.
- Nuts can help, in moderation.
- Drink a glass of carrot juice twice a day.
- Mix one teaspoon each of coriander powder and honey into a glass of water, and drink this paste every morning.
- Cook vegetables with asafoetida and ginger.
- Take no more than ten per cent of your calories from fat (i.e., no more than three-and-a-half ounces of fish, poultry or meat), and no more than five to eight teaspoons of oil a day.
- Lose any excess weight.
- Take morning walks in fresh and clean air (if possible!).
- Do tai chi, yoga, meditation and/or Sudarshan Kriya.

Hypertension / High Blood Pressure

A temporary hike in blood pressure is a common response to an emergency situation, allowing for increased blood supply to the large muscles for a 'fight or flight' reaction. Hypertension is a condition in which the heightened blood pressure does not come down, even after the danger passes. With the smaller blood vessels (arterioles) constricted, carrying less blood to the heart with greater difficulty, the heart gets stuck in emergency mode— a state this muscle is not designed for. Eventually hypertension can result in failure of the heart, brain or kidneys.

Hypertension can be tracked down to fear, anger and so-called Type A characteristics such as striving to achieve too much too early. People who grow up in a tense atmosphere among quarrelsome family members, or are under constant threat to perform well so as to avert the wrath of a demanding parent, or who are constantly made to feel insecure are more prone to hypertension. It can also be triggered or aggravated by problems in adulthood, such as daily skirmishes with a hard-to-please or irrational boss. Often patients are not aware that they are angry or afraid deep within, so their festering emotions just make the problem worse.

If you suffer from hypertension and cannot change your situation, pray for God's help. From time to time ask yourself,

'How am I feeling? Am I happy?' If the answer is no, make two tight fists, try to *feel* your feelings with complete attention, and then imagine letting your feelings go as you loosen your fists.

Having done this, ask yourself, 'What is it that's bothering me? Am I *usually* worried and tense? What can I do about it?' Track down your fears to their source, and think about how you can change your situation to move away from it. If you are not just afraid but angry, think about how to address the problem. If a particular person makes you angry, find a way to talk to him or her about this. Announce calmly that you want to discuss a problem and you would like some help solving it. Do not blame or offend the other person, but try to indicate how his or her behaviour is affecting you adversely.

In one case such a patient determined that he was angry with his boss. The very next day he went to his boss and said politely, 'I know you have many expectations of me, and I may not be able to meet all of them despite trying my best. But I have only one expectation from you: so that we can help you better, please encourage and appreciate us more.' The boss was taken aback, and spent the next half hour expressing his concerns over a cup of tea and assuring his team of more understanding behaviour in future. The patient had such a deep sense of peace and relief after this incident that he surprised his doctors with a dramatic decrease in blood pressure.

Finally, relax more often. Instead of taking pills, take time on a regular basis to slow down, meditate and enjoy being with nature, playing with children or whatever else gives you quiet pleasure. You may decide to practice yoga, especially shavasana or yoga nidra. If applicable, give Reiki to the past moment that caused your present situation, and move on.

Recommended Affirmations: 2, 5–8, 11, 21, 27 and 30

Reiki Positions:

- For both high and low blood pressure: B2–B3, C3, C6 and D5.
- For low blood pressure only: A7 with both hands on the back, and A4–A6.

Dietary and Other Suggestions: See those under 'Stroke', above.

Leukaemia

Originating in the bone marrow, leukaemia is actually a cancer of the blood cells. It causes the overproduction of immature and damaged white blood cells, which then crowd out the red blood cells. There are two kinds of leukaemia: lymphoblastic and myeloid. Symptoms of myeloid leukaemia include a bleeding nose, bleeding gums, bleeding rectum, internal bleeding, pain in the upper abdomen, anaemia, fever and recurring infection. Lymphoblastic leukaemia develops rapidly, presenting the patient with fever, lack of energy, loss of appetite, weight loss, anaemia, headaches, nosebleeds and, for women, excessive menstrual bleeding. Leukaemia of either kind can be acute or chronic, but both show the patient's hopelessness with regard to expressing creativity.

Recommended Affirmations: 2, 6–7, 16, 21–22, 26–27 and 30
Reiki Positions: B1–B7, C1–C7, D5 and D7 with T variation, followed by full-body Reiki with mental healing
Dietary and Other Suggestions:

- Eat plenty of fresh fruits and vegetables, especially citrus fruits, guavas, broccoli, cauliflower, leafy greens, carrots and cabbage, plus whole-grain cereals, wheat germ, brown rice, molasses, nuts, pulses and oily fish.
- Avoid smoking, alcohol and animal fat.

Low Blood Pressure

Low blood pressure indicates an escapist attitude towards your problems: you tend to run away from them rather than accept, confront, examine and solve them. Start accepting yourself as you are, and try to observe the world around you very keenly. If you idly notice that your table is messy without doing anything about it for several days, you will eventually get to a point where you can't think of anything but cleaning it up.

Recommended Affirmations: 8–9, 16, 18–19 and 21
Reiki Positions: C3, C6, D1, D7 and across the shoulder blades.
Dietary and Other Suggestions:

- Eat smaller but more frequent meals.
- Eat more salt.

- Drink plenty of wheat-grass juice.
- Do moderate exercise such as yoga or tai chi.
- Do mental mathematics or solve puzzles.
- Raise the head end of your bed four to six inches.

Mononucleosis

Monocytes are large white blood cells that defend the body by digesting harmful or unwanted matter. In a healthy person, they are few in number; mononucleosis is the presence of too many monocytes in the blood. Symptoms include persistent sore throat, fever, swollen glands and fatigue. The infection may spread to the liver and spleen, possibly resulting in jaundice or tenderness in the abdomen. Metaphysically, 'mono' is caused by resentment at not getting enough attention, love and approval.

Recommended Affirmations: 2, 5–7, 16, 18, 21, 26–27 and 34
Reiki Positions: B1–B7, C3–C7, D5, and ideally full-body treatment with mental healing
Dietary and Other Suggestions:
- Drink lots of fluids, except tea, coffee and cola.
- Do moderate exercise such as yoga, tai chi or simply walking (not running).
- Get lots of rest.

Oedema

Oedema is a condition caused by the leakage of extra watery fluid from the blood into the body's tissues and cavities. Usually experienced as puffiness in the feet, ankles, eyes and lungs, it indicates an unconscious tendency to hold on to things (or people) too tightly. Remember that holding on to something is precisely what makes it hard to continue possessing it. Loosen your grip on anything if you want to see it come back to you.

Recommended Affirmations: 7
Reiki Positions: A5, B1, B3, B6–B7, C3–C4, C6–C7 and D5.
Dietary and Other Suggestions:
- Eat plenty of nuts, dried fruits, pulses, whole grains, avocados, tomatoes, potatoes, bananas and oranges (sources of potassium).

- Take a pinch of ground broom seeds with a teaspoon of honey once a day.
- Cut out salt from your diet. Avoid smoked foods, tinned or dried soups and foods with additives.
- Lose any excess weight.
- Do moderate exercise such as yoga, tai chi or simply walking (not running).

Thrombosis

Thrombosis is the presence of blood clots in the vascular system. Clots may form due to cholesterol containing masses known as plaques in the vessel walls. The plaques provide a rough surface where platelets can adhere and form clots. The clot (thrombus) may damage the tissues by cutting off their blood supply, and if it gets dislodged it can travel down to smaller vessels and block the blood supply to vital organs. Thrombosis can manifest itself as thrombophlebitis (legs), myocardial infarction (heart attack), stroke (brain), pulmonary embolism (lungs) and coronary thrombosis (heart).

Thrombosis generally indicates a stagnancy, immobility or rigidity in the patient's life. Letting go of rigidly held views and beliefs will have a positive effect on your health. Coronary thrombosis indicates loneliness, fear and a feeling of self-disapproval; the patient does not consider her- or himself a success.

Recommended Affirmations: 4, 6–7 and 28
Reiki Positions: B1–B6, C3–C4, C6–C7 and D5 and the affected area.

Dietary and Other Suggestions:

- Eat more substances that act as coagulants—peppers, pineapples, melons, eggplant, garlic, onions, ginger, olive oil.
- Eat more turnips, oranges, parsley, watercress, asparagus, carrots, green pepper and spinach, preferably in juice form.
- Eat plenty of oat bran and pulses.
- Avoid margarine and all saturated fats—animal proteins, dairy products, coconut oil—as these are instrumental in

clotting. You can eat oily fishes such as herring, trout and mackerel.

- Replace white sugar with honey or jaggery powder, and use even that sparingly. Sugar adds to the 'sticking' tendency of the platelets.
- Cut out salt and smoking.
- Red wine may help, if you stick to less than two glasses a day. Give the wine Reiki before you drink it.

THE DIGESTIVE SYSTEM

The stomach receives and digests not only food but whatever we perceive, think and experience. Whenever fear or any similar emotion gets in the way of our digesting a new idea or situation, our stomach gets upset. Rejection, disappointment, rejection of our own feelings, and fear of disapproval by someone whose opinion is important to you can all result in stomach aches. When we feel secure and trust ourselves, we experience and assimilate our feelings and conflicts properly.

Appetite Loss

The appetite is controlled through the appestat, a part of the brain that evaluates the body's needs and signals hunger through hormones. Malfunctioning of the appestat can make a well-fed person feel hungry and a hungry person feel satisfied. The common cold, travel sickness, indigestion, depression, worry and improper diet can all bring down the appetite temporarily. Loss of appetite suggests that one has accumulated a great deal of fear, and one resists the idea of accepting oneself. One may go so far as to hate oneself, feeling that one is unworthy.

Recommended Affirmations: 14, 19 and 28

Reiki Positions: B1–B7

Dietary and Other Suggestions:

- Squeeze the juice of a lemon into a glass of water, sweeten it with honey and drink it every morning.
- Drink two tablespoons of wheat-grass juice thrice a day and two teaspoons of coriander juice twice a day.

- Eat plenty of bananas and other fresh fruits, potatoes and other vegetables, nuts, seeds (especially pumpkin seeds) and whole grains.
- Cut down on bran, salt, alcohol, tea, coffee and chocolate.
- Avoid vitamin D or iron supplements unless a doctor prescribes them.

Constipation / Colon Problems

Constipation and colon problems stem from a fear of releasing old ideas, thoughts, attitudes and repressed negative feelings— a refusal to let go of the past. Stinginess and excessive frugality can also contribute to the problem. Wearing old clothes so as to preserve new ones as long as possible, over-using your toothbrush, getting attached to your meaningless but secure job . . . all show a complete distrust in God's plan for you. A river may not know what lies ahead, but it knows that wherever it goes it will find a bank on either side. Do not attempt to hoard or hold on to things you do not use, things that have outlived their utility. Do not carry with you in life what needs to be left behind.

Recommended Affirmations: 1, 4, 6–7, 16 and 24
Reiki Positions: A5, B2-B7 (with emphasis on B2 and B6), D6–D7 and position with one hand under the back of the neck and the other at B6 (below the navel).

Dietary and Other Suggestions:

- Switch to a wholesome vegetarian diet. Increase your fibre intake by adding barley to all vegetable soups and eating whole-grain cereals.
- Sprinkle bran over all your food. Do not try to get all your fibre from bran, however, as it may interfere with the absorption of iron and calcium. Limit its use to two or three teaspoons per meal and increase it only cautiously.
- Eat plenty of apples, prunes, apricots, raisins, peaches, pears with the skin, nuts, dried beans, figs, raisins, popcorn and oatmeal.
- Drink ten to twelve glasses of water every day.
- Drink half a glass of spinach juice every morning.

- Have some guava or papaya before each meal.
- Eat some tomatoes or drink tomato juice with every meal.
- Grind two parts psyllium seeds with one part flux and one part oat bran, add water, and drink the mixture an hour before your bedtime.
- Squeeze the juice of one lemon (or take one teaspoon of powdered gooseberries), stir it into a glass of warm water and drink it before you go to bed.
- Avoid coffee, chocolate, tea, cola and white bread (replace with whole-grain bread).
- Drink alcohol in moderation—less than two glasses a day.
- Stop smoking.
- Do some physical exercise every day.
- Do not suppress the need to answer nature's call. The longer digested food stays in your bowel system, the drier it gets, and the more difficult it becomes to pass it. Train yourself to visit the toilet after every meal, not just when it's convenient.
- Chew your food well, especially nuts and seeds.
- Do yoga, Surya Namaskar and/or tai chi.

Diabetes Mellitus

Insulin is a hormone produced by the pancreas to keep the optimal glucose (sugar) level in the bloodstream. Too much glucose in the blood because of inadequate insulin results in a disease called diabetes mellitus or simply diabetes. Symptoms include thirst, frequent urination, weight loss, fatigue, recurrent infection, vision problems and slow healing of wounds. Diabetics are at risk for heart disease, kidney problems, atherosclerosis, nerve damage, infection and even blindness. Nutrition, weight control, regular rhythmic exercise and above all a positive attitude must all be embraced.

At the emotional level, the pancreas represents sweetness in one's life. Diabetes tends to afflict people who yearn for love but do not allow themselves to be loved. They either doubt the love of others, or they take it for granted. The pancreas can also be affected by a desire to control everything and everyone around you—insisting that people behave the way *you* want them to; being intolerant of ideas different from your own; pitying yourself too much, comparing your life with what you think should have been; aiming to catch others doing things wrong rather than encouraging them to do things right. When you squeeze joy, fun, love and sweetness out of your life, you are on your way to attracting diabetes. Generally speaking, a difficult relationship with one's mother (often unknown at the conscious level) affects those organs energized by the third chakra on the left side of the body, including the pancreas.

Recommended Affirmations: 5, 7–9, 11–13, 16–19, 21 and 35

Reiki Positions: If you are already on insulin, watch its level closely—Reiki usually results in a drastic drop in the need for insulin.

- A1, A5, A7 (with both hands at the back), B1(T variation), B3, B5, B7, C3, C6, D5, D7 and the elbow tips.
- For deteriorating eyesight, A1–A3 and B7 for females, D7 for males.

Dietary and Other Suggestions:

- Mix the juice of a mango with that of blueberries and drink it daily. Mix the juice of fresh gooseberries with honey and take that regularly as well. Excess mango consumption is not recommended.
- Mix two parts carrot juice with one part spinach juice and drink the mixture daily.
- Drink the juice of a bitter gourd diluted with water six times its quantity thrice for four months.
- Eat preparations of turnip, fenugreek or bitter gourd with gram-flour bread.
- Eat plenty of fresh fruit (except grapes and mangoes, which have too much sugar) and vegetables, especially onions. Eat plenty of garlic. Drink plenty of vegetable (not fruit) juices.
- Avoid sugar. Adopt a high-carbonate plant-fibre diet high in starch and fibre (whole-grain bread, beans, soybeans, peas, lentils; at least seventy per cent of your total intake) but low in proteins (meat, cheese and eggs; not more than twenty per cent) and fat (not more than ten per cent).

- If you eat fish, limit it to once a week, and choose varieties low in oil and high in fat. Stick to regular mealtimes.
- Cut down on sweetened soft drinks, chocolate, biscuits, sweets and cakes.
- Avoid artificial sweeteners; they pose various possible health risks.
- Cut out alcohol.
- Avoid heavy meals and tinned, smoked, processed, salty, fried and fatty foods.
- Lose any excess weight.
- For relaxation and stress reduction, try yoga nidra, meditation, and/or vipasana. Some people claim to have recovered permanently from mild diabetes through vipasana and Reiki. Regular tai chi, slow Surya Namaskar, yogasanas and half an hour of brisk walking, cycling or swimming are some other recommended exercises. Avoid strenuous exercises or over-exertion.

Diarrhoea

Diarrhoea is an inflammation of the large intestine. It normally lasts just a day or two; seek immediate medical assistance if it lasts longer. When you refuse to register or assimilate an experience, hoping it will pass quickly through your life because you find it frightening or overwhelming, your body correspondingly refuses to assimilate what you eat. Diarrhoea can also be the result of hopelessness, fear of rejection, attempts to get over something quickly without consciously feeling it, and long-term simmering aggression and anger. All experiences come to you when and because you need them, so do not try to bypass them. By the same token, do not try to stop diarrhoea—interfering with this natural detoxification process may complicate matters and result in secondary problems.

Recommended Affirmations: 5 and 16

Reiki Positions: A4–A5, B—B3, B5–B7, C4, C7, insides of the calves, and D4–D7.

Dietary and Other Suggestions:

- Cut out solid foods for a day or two. Drink only apple juice or mineral water every half hour. Alternately, stir one teaspoon of salt and then 8 teaspoons of sugar in one litre of boiled water (or in half a litre of orange juice). When diarrhoea subsides start eating boiled white rice, dry white toast, carrots, and vegetable soups or juices.

- One day after the diarrhoea subsides, start eating more solids such as steamed carrots and bananas.
- Start taking yoghurt or buttermilk with a pinch of salt thrice a day after three days of diarrhoea.
- Mix a dash each of powdered cinnamon, dry ginger, saffron and crushed caraway seeds with half a teaspoon of garlic juice and take it twice a day.
- Some people are lactose-intolerant. If you have diarrhoea frequently, give up milk products (except yoghurt and buttermilk) and see if that helps.
- During diarrhoea, cut out carbonated drinks, alcohol, coffee, beans, Brussels sprouts, cabbage, bread and pasta.

Dysentery

Dysentery, an infection of the bowels, has two forms: amoebic and bacillary. Both are caused and aggravated by poor hygiene and/or contaminated food or water. The patient feels feverish, experiences gas and vomiting, and may suffer from abdominal cramps and diarrhoea. Amoebic dysentery is often accompanied by blood, mucous or pus in the ill-formed stools.

Amoebic dysentery shows a fear that others are determined to harm one. Bacillary dysentery shows a feeling of being exploited by others, or of general helplessness.

Recommended Affirmations: 5, 7, 16, 18–19, 21–23, 26–27 and 29–30

Reiki Positions: Ten minutes at B2–B3 and B5–B6 thrice a day until the dysentery is cured.

Dietary and Other Suggestions:
- Eat nothing but apples with skin for three days, up to ten a day.
- After the first week, eat only cooked food.
- Peel your fruits, even though under normal circumstances

you should eat them with their skin.

- To compensate for the loss of minerals and salts passing out through the stool, eat more soup and drink more vegetable juices and clean water, taken with salt (or simply take an electrolyte).
- Avoid solid foods. Eat bland meals such as plain, parboiled whole rice.
- Give up dairy and animal products until three weeks after the diarrhoea stops.
- Make a paste with some basil leaves, fenugreek leaves (or powder), a few drops of lemon juice, powdered black pepper, roasted caraway powder, aniseed, coriander powder and three teaspoons of honey, and take it thrice a day.

Flatulence

Flatulence is the formation of excessive gas or wind due to the swallowing of air along with hurriedly gulped food. It can also be caused by carbonated drinks, or simply by the failure of the digestive system to break down certain foods, in which case the remaining residues ferment and rot. Beans, broccoli, cauliflower, cucumbers, capsicums, lettuce, nuts, onions, peas, radishes, apples, melons and prunes can all be difficult to digest. Flatulence manifests itself in frequent belching, passing of wind and constipation.

Trying to do too many things indiscriminately, without understanding your real needs, may result in flatulence. Take on only what you can handle, in harmony with your temperament. Accept yourself as you are, with all your limitations, and learn to refuse what you do not want. Flatulence may also occur when you are unable to swallow something and try to compensate by swallowing air with your food.

Recommended Affirmations: 21, 26–27 and 29–30

Reiki Positions: A4–A5, B2–B6, C2, C4–C5, C7, D5 and across the shoulders.

Dietary and Other Suggestions:

- Alternate hot and cold compresses on the abdomen.
- Sit erect while eating.

- Eat more garlic, peppermint and live yoghurt.
- Cut down on pulses (peas, beans, lentils, cabbages) or use spices that aid in digesting them, such as ginger and coriander.
- Do not eat starches and proteins together.
- If you suffer from constipation, increase your intake of high-fibre foods only gradually.
- Make liberal use of lemon balm, rosemary, sage, thyme, summer savoury, caraway and fennel seeds.
- Avoid heavy meals and do not overeat. Eat slowly and consciously. Sip liquids rather than gulp them. Before you drink a fizzy drink, let the bubbles escape.
- Drink mint or fennel tea after each meal.
- Keep a diary of foods eaten and the extent of ensuing discomfort to find out what is it that troubles you. Then you can avoid it.

Food Poisoning

Germs that inflame the linings of the stomach and intestines can be picked up from reheated or undercooked food, an unhygienic kitchen or contaminated milk, fish or poultry. Nausea, vomiting, diarrhoea, abdominal cramps, fever and sweating are some of the symptoms. Food poisoning afflicts those who let others control their lives, resulting in a feeling of vulnerability.

Recommended Affirmations: 5, 7, 22–23, 29 and 35
Reiki Positions: B2–B7, C4, C7 and D5–D7
Dietary and Other Suggestions
   Preventive:

- Always wash your hands with soap before handling food and starting meals, and after using the toilet.
- Keep your kitchen sparklingly clean. Ensure that it's well ventilated, equipped with exhaust fans or chimneys. Wash dishes thoroughly, taking care to rinse the soap off completely.
- Throw kitchen waste only in a covered bin, which should be kept well away from all fresh food items.

- Avoid meat if possible. If you must eat it, keep raw meat away from cooked meat. Wash your hands thoroughly after handling raw meat.
- Never reheat cooked food.
- The usual sources of food poisoning are seafood, soft-rinded cheese, unwashed salad, pork, beef, poultry, eggs and sweets, usually because they have not been kept or prepared with proper hygiene. (Vegetarians have an advantage here.)
- Do not keep cooked dishes warm over very low heat, as bacteria multiply quickly in warm settings.

Theraupetic:
- Eat plenty of unpeeled fresh fruits.
- After the diarrhoea or vomiting ends, resume eating only easily digestible foods such as cereals, puddings and broth. Avoid high-fibre, spicy, acidic, greasy, dairy and very sweet foods for at least two days. Avoid all solid food, and replace fluid loss by taking an electrolyte solution and diluted fruit juice with salt and honey at regular intervals throughout the day. You may also take plain apple juice.
- Take a teaspoon of garlic juice thrice a day.
- Cut down on refined carbohydrates, deep-fried fatty foods and alcohol.

Gallstones

Gallstones are dense lumps of cholesterol, calcium deposits and bile pigments that crystallize to form stones in the gall bladder or bile ducts. Unease, discomfort or severe pain in the upper abdomen (sometimes accompanied by vomiting), especially after heavy or fatty meals, may indicate the presence of gallstones. In extreme cases, surgery may be required to remove the stones or the gall bladder itself.

Gall-bladder problems represent accumulated anger or aggression, whether expressed or unexpressed. Gallstones indicate the bitter residue of past experiences involving humiliation, anger, grudges and the acute inability to forgive others. Be attentive to all that makes you angry.

Recommended Affirmations: 2, 7–9, 12, 16, 18–19, 21, 26, 28 and 35

Reiki Positions: Several long applications on B3, B5 and D5.

Dietary and Other Suggestions:

- Cut out dairy products and animal fats.
- Stick to a diet low in fat and high in soluble fibre (from oat bran and pulses) and starch.
- Eat plenty of whole grains and fresh vegetables (have a salad with every meal), take plenty of fresh lemon juice and cook with polyunsaturated oils such as sunflower and safflower.
- Avoid fried and fatty foods.
- Lose any excess weight.
- You can take coffee, chocolate and alcohol in moderation.
- European artichokes have been found useful in the treatment of gallstones.

Gastritis

Gastritis is an inflammation of the stomach lining. It manifests itself in a burning sensation between the top of the stomach and the chest; heartburn; nausea; and flatulence. It can be caused by excess alcohol, the use of anti-inflammatory drugs for arthritis, and the consumption of rich and spicy foods too late at night. Metaphysically, it may stem from constant, prolonged stress, worry and anxiety.

Recommended Affirmations: 16, 22 and 25–27

Reiki Positions: B2–B4, B6, C4, C7 and D4.

Dietary and Other Suggestions:

- Drink ten to twelve glasses of water every day.
- Eat plenty of bananas and apples.
- Eat boiled white rice for the first two days. Return to a normal diet only gradually.
- See suggestions given for heartburn and indigestion/belching, below.

Heartburn

Heartburn occurs when you repeatedly have to swallow your anger. Learn to communicate your annoyance in a positive way.

Recommended Affirmations: 16, 21–25

Reiki Positions: Ten minutes twice daily on A1, A4–A5, B2–B3, B5–B7 and the outside of the upper arms. If the problem is severe, add A4, C4, C7 and the afflicted spot for at least five minutes each.

Dietary and Other Suggestions:

- Hot compresses over the stomach area may help. Relax your muscles to improve the blood supply there.
- Eat slowly and consciously. Take small bites and chew each mouthful well, focusing on the taste. Eat smaller meals more often.
- Cook with ginger.
- Avoid tight belts or girdles; use suspenders instead. To lift a heavy object, use your knees to bend down, not your spine.
- Eat your dinner at least 2½ hours before bedtime.
- Raise the head end of your bed four to six inches.
- Avoid milk (decline the advice of those who recommend it for ulcers and heartburn), cheese and other dairy products, tomatoes, alcohol, fried and fatty foods, meat, coffee, tea, cola and chocolates.
- Stop smoking.
- See other suggestions under 'Ulcers.'

Hemorrhoids (Piles)

When a nerve around the anus ruptures, blood collects in a weaker part of the vein wall, causing it to swell and become itchy and painful. Prolonged tension in this area interferes with circulation and can eventually force the blood backwards into a vein that swells up and finally ruptures. All this has to do with your tightening the muscles around your anus because of unconscious stress in your life. The physical causes of hemorrhoids are a sedentary job (involving a lot of sitting), an unwholesome diet, frequent and prolonged constipation and general disharmony in one's attitude towards life. Obesity intensifies the problem. The emotional reasons for piles are similar to those for constipation: general stress, fear of not meeting targets or deadlines, inability to forgive oneself and others and unwillingness to let go of a stressful or threatening situation. An abscess here wants to draw your attention to the anger stemming from the conflict between a need to let go and a desire to continue to cling to some aspect of your life. (See also 'Abscess' in 'The Skin', below.)

While hemorrhoidal bleeding shows anger, disappointment and frustration, itching reflects guilt and remorse over an unpleasant past experience. Remember to love yourself, and maintain balance in your life by refusing unreasonable deadlines and taking life easy. Think about what might be troubling you; then consider and begin implementing solutions. Draw the appropriate lessons from this stressful situation, and use them to avoid such situations in the future.

Recommended Affirmations: 7

Reiki Positions:

- Five minutes each at B2–B3, B5–B7, C2–C3, C5–C6, D1, D5 and the soles of the feet, excluding the heel.
- D7 for half an hour. Place the middle finger over the anal opening and place the other hand on the tailbone. (Use basic D7 if the patient is other than yourself or your spouse/ partner.)
- Beneath the coccyx to the perineum.
- Both hands on the fold of the buttocks.

Dietary and Other Suggestions:

- Avoid alcohol, smoking, coffee, peppermint drinks and hot, spicy food such as curries.
- Eat one or two tomatoes with every meal. Eat some yoghurt and one clove of garlic each day. Take fifty grams of black sesame seeds with yogurt.
- Adopt a high-fiber diet with foods such as linseed, whole-meal bread and brown rice. (Cut down on refined carbohydrates.) Eat plenty of apples, pears, beans, oats, and cooked leafy green vegetables. Patients with persistent hemorrhoids also need plenty of pulses, nuts, dark-green vegetables and fresh fruits.
- Eat two guavas with a few basil leaves on an empty stomach every morning.
- Drink lots of fluids, including fruit and vegetable juices and

ten to twelve glasses of water daily.
- Every night, drink a glass of buttermilk with a bit of rock salt, one teaspoon of roasted cumin seed and 1 teaspoon thymol (*ajwaaeen*).
- Alternate hot and cold packs on the affected area.
- Apply a paste of basil leaves and some sesame or castor oil to the affected area daily.
- Lose any excess weight.
- Apply talcum powder to the affected area after your bath. Do not scratch.
- A simple exercise can help: stand with your feet a few inches apart and your legs slightly bent at the knee. Pat your left buttock and then your right, just to make sure they're loose. Pause for a bit, then repeat. Between each two sets of patting, imagine and feel that the buttocks are getting more and more relaxed. Do this six times.

Hernia

A hernia is a protrusion of an organ in the abdominal region due to a localized weakness of muscles. Inguinal hernia involves the groin area, while hiatus hernia affects the spot where the oesophagus meets the diaphragm. Both cause acidic juices to flow back into the oesophagus, causing heartburn, indigestion, gas or general discomfort.

Often, however, hernias have no symptoms at all. A hernia asks you to look within to see whether stress is making you hostile and harsh towards yourself. Remember that you do not need to prove yourself to others; you are already a unique expression of the Latent Oneness. Accept yourself and live life unconditionally with complete trust, respect and love. Learn to nurture those relationships that have gone sour, establish rational priorities, relieve yourself of unnecessary stress and learn to express yourself in more positive ways.

Recommended Affirmations: 7, 16, 22–23, 25–29
Reiki Positions: B2, D4 and directly on the hernia.
Dietary and Other Suggestions:
- Wash the affected area locally with coffee.

- Cook with herbs such as dill, fennel, mint (not peppermint), rosemary, sage and tarragon to improve digestion. Avoid fried, fatty and spicy foods.
- Avoid very hot or cold foods and fizzy drinks.
- Eat smaller meals more often. Avoid large meals, especially at night; finish your last meal two to three hours before bedtime.
- Stop smoking.
- Raise the head end of your bed four to six inches.
- Follow the suggestions under 'Heartburn', above.

Hypoglycaemia

Hypoglycaemia, or low blood sugar, can be indicated by hunger, fatigue, weakness, cold sweats, palpitations, dizziness and/or a confused state of mind. The patient may even fall unconscious. Diabetics are prone to hypoglycaemia, as their bodies find it difficult to regulate the level of sugar in the blood. Metaphysical causes are the same as those for diabetes.

Recommended Affirmations: 5, 7–9, 11–13, 16–19, 21 and 35

Reiki Positions: If you are already on insulin, watch its level closely, as Reiki usually results in a drastic drop in the need for insulin.

- A1, A5, A7 (with both hands at the back), B1(T variation), B3, B5, B7, C3, C6, D5, D7 and the elbow tips.
- For deteriorating eyesight, A1–A3 and B7 for females, D7 for males.

Dietary and Other Suggestions:

- Eat whole grains, pulses, potatoes (with the skin) and pasta. Eat fresh fruits, dried fruits and honey only in moderation.
- Eat more proteins, as they take longer to digest and help prevent drops in blood sugar.
- Keep regular mealtimes. Eat smaller meals more often.

Indigestion

Stress, eating too quickly, overeating, eating too much rich or fatty food, smoking, alcohol, coffee, and certain medicines such as aspirin can all cause indigestion, which manifests itself as belching, gas, abdominal pain, heartburn, wind, a bloated feeling, nausea and/or regurgitation. Indigestion can also result from the inability of the system to break down certain foods such as beans, broccoli, cabbage, cauliflower, cucumbers, capsicums, unripe fruits, lettuce, radishes, onions, peas, nuts, melons, prunes or cheese, which leave residues that ferment in the bowels. See if you can figure out which foods aggravate the condition, and avoid them.

Metaphysically, indigestion results when you nag a lot, always finding something to complain about, or from a looming fear that something bad is about to happen to you. Belching, specifically, shows a rush to digest things without experiencing their taste fully. What you need is peace—not pace. Give complete attention and time to everything you do, especially eating.

Recommended Affirmations: 2, 4, 7, 9, 11, 16, 22, 25 and 35
Reiki Positions: Ten minutes twice daily at A4–A5, B1–B3, B5–B7. If the problem is severe, add five minutes at C2–C5, C7, D1 and D5–D7.

Dietary and Other Suggestions:

- Drink plenty of papaya and pineapple juice.
- Half an hour before each meal, drink a glass of water with some lemon juice, or some grated ginger in lemon juice.
- Rest for ten to thirty minutes before and after each meal.
- Take a little asafoetida, about the size of a millet grain, with a banana once a day.
- When your stomach is upset, take watercress.
- Follow the suggestions under 'Heartburn', above.
- Eat plenty of fibre-rich foods such as whole-meal bread and brown rice.
- Drink ten to twelve glasses of water every day, but not within half an hour of a meal (or with a meal).
- Eat smaller meals more often.
- Cut down on alcohol, coffee, tea, pickles, vinegar, ice cream, fried, fatty and spicy foods (especially late at night), cola, beer and chewing gum.
- Stop smoking.
- Keep your mouth closed while eating.

- Do not drink through straws or from cans or bottles.
- Be aware of the present moment. Make a running mental commentary on what you are doing, especially when you eat, as in: 'I have torn a little piece from the bread, have taken a small morsel of vegetables and am bringing it to my mouth. I am chewing it now, slowly and carefully. It tastes nice. I am still chewing it, still enjoying it. I have chewed it so well that it has almost become a paste. Now I am swallowing, and it is going down my throat to nourish my body. Now I am taking a second morsel . . . '
- Avoid gossip, anger, sarcasm and emotionally unpleasant situations.
- Optional: do yoga and meditation every day.

Intestinal Cramps

Abdominal pain represents anguish over what we see around us, or fear of failure in some important aspect of life. It tells us to let go of certain phases of life that are no longer required for one's personal growth. On the emotional level, judging, evaluation, criticism and assimilation of impressions is the small intestine's job—so when you feel materially insecure and find lots of things to criticize, your intestines find it difficult to assimilate food as well. Don't worry about small things—and learn to see everything in life as a small thing. Go on a 'fast' once a week when you do not judge or criticize anyone or anything.

Recommended Affirmations: 16, 22–23 and 26–27
Reiki Positions: B2–B4, B6, C4, C7 and D4.
Dietary and Other Suggestions:

- Eat plenty of whole grains, fruits and vegetables. Add bran to your diet very gradually.
- If you are sensitive to gas-producing foods such as beans, cabbage, Brussels sprouts, broccoli, cauliflower and onions, eat them with caution. If they bother you, mix a teaspoon each of aniseed, caraway and fennel in a cup of boiling water, strain the mixture and drink it hot.
- Mix two teaspoons each of lemon juice, mint juice and ginger

juice with honey and take the mixture when cramps strike.
- Stir half a teaspoon each of garlic, basil and coriander-leaf juice and a pinch of black salt in four teaspoons of water and take the mixture.
- Mix roasted asafoetida and caraway with a bit of black salt and dry ginger, and take it with a spoonful of warm water.
- Roast and grind caraway seeds, and take them with a spoonful of honey after each meal.
- Stick to regular mealtimes.
- Cut out fats, heavy sauces, fried foods, salad oils and dairy products.
- Drink lots of fluids, including ten to twelve glasses of water every day. Avoid tea, coffee, cola and chocolate.
- When cramps strike, place a hot-water bottle on your abdomen.

Nausea/Vomiting

The sickly, uncomfortable feeling of needing to vomit is known as nausea. It may or may not be accompanied by actual vomiting. Nausea can result from overeating, morning sickness, motion sickness, migraines, vertigo, food poisoning, gastroenteritis or uncontrolled diabetes. A reflection of our fear and consequent desire to reject an idea or experience, it is the body's way of saying, 'No more!' When we cannot digest something, physically or mentally, our body throws it up. Vomiting may even take place in response to an unexpected success or happiness—an experience too rich to be swallowed. Such elation is sometimes hidden under an apparent feeling of sadness in order to conform to social expectations; for example, the death of a close relative may relieve you of some unpleasant responsibilities.

Recommended Affirmations: 5, 7–9, 12, 16, 18, 21, 22, 24 and 25

Reiki Positions: A5, B2–B6, C4, C7 and D5. The patient may vomit in order to detoxify. This is fine.

Dietary and Other Suggestions:
- Take one or two teaspoons of ginger juice (you can mix onion juice in it too) or peppermint or lemon or basil or

coriander leaves.

- Once the vomiting is over, eat vegetable soups, boiled whole-grain unpolished rice and whole-wheat bread before gradually resuming your normal diet.
- Boil four cloves in a cup of water until the water is half evaporated. Filter this water through a sieve, sweeten it with a teaspoon of honey and drink it. Lie down on your left side and try to get some sleep.
- Drink watermelon juice sweetened with honey every morning.
- Chew a few black peppercorns.
- Hold the web between your thumb and index finger and massage it with deep pressure. Do the same to the tendons between your second and third toes.
- Sip liquids rather than gulp them. Before you drink a fizzy drink, let the bubbles escape.

THE LIVER

The liver is located on the upper right-hand side of the body, just below the diaphragm, between the ribs and pelvis. It carries out almost five hundred tasks, many of which are crucial for life itself. Most important, the liver produces bile (to disintegrate fats in the duodenum); stores carbohydrates and a variety of vitamins and minerals; controls blood-sugar levels; converts ammonia into urea and proteins; and removes toxins or whatever is not good for the body. On the emotional or spiritual level, therefore, it reflects on moderation versus excess: for example, you may be focusing on one aspect of life to the exclusion of other important areas, or you may be carrying ideals too lofty to be practical in your life, leaving you forever dissatisfied or guilty. The liver also manifests our level of spiritual evolution, the way we live our life. If we are slow to make important decisions and implement them, or if we fear moving ahead, the liver does likewise—it gets sluggish. Cases of extreme bias, skewed reasoning and prejudice may result in jaundice.

Hepatitis

Hepatitis is an inflammation of the liver, usually marked by fever and jaundice. It reminds us to liberate ourselves from negative emotions stemming from extreme mental conflict, resistance to change, fear, anger and hatred before the problem escalates to its next level—cirrhosis of the liver.

Recommended Affirmations: 2, 4, 7–9, 11–12, 16, 21–22, 25 and 35

Reiki Positions: D7, C6 and across the shoulder blades.

Dietary and Other Suggestions:

- Drink fresh fruit and vegetable juices and soups every day.
- Avoid fatty foods and alcohol.
- Do some yogic exercise.
- Place cold packs on the abdomen.
- Follow the suggestions under 'Jaundice', below.

Jaundice

Jaundice is a liver disorder marked by a yellowing of the skin and eyes. When gallstones or a liver disorder obstruct the bile duct, the yellow pigment called bilirubin comes directly into the bloodstream. Haemolytic jaundice results from the breakdown of red blood cells. Liver-cell jaundice results from hepatitis or from cirrhosis/liver failure. Though jaundice usually indicates Hepatitis A, from which patients normally recover within three weeks, it can also indicate serious liver problems such as cancer, cirrhosis or Hepatitis B.

Recommended Affirmations: 5–6, 8, 11–12, 16, 21, 25, 28, 30 and 34–35

Reiki Positions: A1–A5, B2–B3, B5–B6, C4, C7 and across the shoulder blades.

Dietary and Other Suggestions:

- Avoid fats and alcohol. Cut down on spicy, fried and fatty foods, coffee, tea and chocolate.
- Drink plenty of fresh vegetable juices such as celery or carrot. Watercress is also beneficial.
- Eat more prunes, muskmelon, papayas, strawberries, watercress, dried apricots, leafy green vegetables, soybeans,

green cabbage, pulses, oats, unsweetened muesli, whole-meal bread, brown rice, wheat germ, yeast extract and nuts.

- Drink a glass of tomato or cauliflower juice mixed with carrot juice twice or thrice a day.
- Mix jaggery powder and turmeric powder in half a cup of white onion juice and take it in the morning and evening.
- Mash four cloves of garlic and mix them into half a cup of hot milk, then drink more milk. Try this for a week.
- Drink a glass of bitter-gourd juice in the morning and evening.
- Eat a handful of barley, and then drink some fresh, clean sugarcane juice.
- Take two teaspoons of honey thrice a day.

Parasites

Discomfort and itching in an otherwise healthy bottom may be caused by parasites; red and black stools definitely are. Parasites come into being when you refuse to take charge of your life, preferring others to run it for you. Stop depending on others—take your life back into your own hands.

Recommended Affirmations: 29
Reiki Positions: B2–B3, B5–B6, C4, C7 and D5
Dietary and Other Suggestions:

- To *prevent* parasites, follow the suggestions given under 'Food Poisoning', above.
- Mash dry lemon or papaya seeds into a powder and take half a teaspoon with a quarter cup of water every day for a week.
- Mix some lemon (or gooseberry or pomegranate or mint) juice into a glass of water and drink it on an empty stomach.
- On an empty stomach, drink some coconut water and eat some raw coconut.
- On an empty stomach, drink carrot juice or buttermilk with a bit of black pepper.
- On an empty stomach, eat some tomato with black pepper and black salt.
- For children: on an empty stomach, eat two walnuts and

then drink some milk.

- Take one teaspoon of onion or garlic juice every two hours until symptoms disappear.
- Take three garlic cloves with some honey thrice a day for two months.
- Every night for a week, eat two apples before you go to bed. Do not drink any water after this.

Tapeworms/Threadworms

The ribbon-like tapeworm, which can be anywhere from a few millimetres to ten metres long, finds its way into the intestines through contaminated food, usually beef or pork. The resulting infection caused manifests itself as nausea, diarrhoea and general abdominal discomfort. Metaphysically, tapeworms may present themselves as a result of lack of self-esteem, or specifically a feeling of being dirty or being a victim.

Threadworms, each about a centimetre long, can infect the large intestine and cause inflammation and itching around the anus, plus abdominal pain or bloody vaginal discharge in females. Scratching the itchy anus can reinfect others through the fingernails.

Recommended Affirmations: 2, 5, 8–9, 12, 16 , 21, 25–27, 29–30 and 34

Reiki Positions: B2–B4 and B6, plus mental healing with the intention of getting rid of the worms and clearing away the infection.

Dietary and Other Suggestions:

- Garlic, carrots and pumpkin seeds help in overcoming the infection.
- Keep your fingernails short.
- Stay well away from uncooked beef or pork.
- Always wash your hands with soap before handling food, before starting meals and after using the toilet.
- Keep your kitchen sparklingly clean. Ensure that it's well ventilated, equipped with exhaust fans or chimneys. Wash dishes thoroughly, taking care to rinse the soap off completely.

- Throw kitchen waste only in a covered bin, which should be kept well away from all fresh food items.
- If you must eat meat, keep raw meat away from cooked meat. Wash your hands thoroughly after handling raw meat.
- Never reheat cooked food.

For stubborn tapeworms:

- Fast for twelve hours.
- Remove the skins from sixty grams of pumpkins seeds, grind the pulp to a paste and drink it with a little milk thrice a day.
- Take four teaspoons of castor oil with a cup of fruit juice. The tapeworm may pass out three hours later.

Ulcers

Ulcers are commonly found in the intestinal lining or the first part of the duodenum. Stomach secretions contain pepsin, an enzyme that accelerates the disintegration of proteins and gastric juice (which is mainly hydrochloric acid). Normally the stomach protects itself from these secretions, but when part of the stomach's lining is injured, the tissue in that area gets 'digested' by acids and enzymes, resulting in a depression or hole there. Ulcers afflict those who are frustrated and do not express their feelings well. When we understand and trust that every aspect of our lives has a purpose, we can accept and assimilate our feelings. This obviates the necessity for the stomach to manifest these feelings—especially aggression—in the form of ulcers in order to get noticed. Low self-esteem can also result in ulcers.

Recommended Affirmations: 5–7, 12, 21, 25 and 28

Reiki Positions:

- Ten minutes twice daily on A1, A4–A5, B2–B3, B5–B7 and the outside of the upper arms.
- In severe cases, add at least five minutes at A4, C4, C7 and the afflicted area.

Dietary and Other Suggestions:

- Consume plenty of ginger, spinach, carrots and onions, preferably in juice form. Bananas have also been found to protect the stomach lining.
- Drink a glass of fresh cabbage juice with every meal for two

weeks. Do not heat the juice, mix it with other food or take it on an empty stomach.

- Stick to a wholesome, fibre-rich diet including plenty of yoghurt.
- Cut out smoking (it makes ulcers difficult to heal), alcohol, refined sugar, refined flour, junk food generally, apples, spicy and fried foods, salt, soya sauce, cola, milk, tea and coffee.
- Do not take aspirin, anti-inflammatory drugs or iron supplements, especially on an empty stomach.
- Try stress reduction through yoga, meditation, Sudarshan Kriya, tai chi or yoga nidra. Sleep at least eight or nine hours every night.
- Eat smaller meals more often (say, six instead of three).
- Avoid keeping a cat, as they carry the bacterium 'Helicobacter pylori', which has been found in the stomachs of ulcer patients.

THE SKELETAL/MOTOR SYSTEM

Bones represent stability, support and the norms we choose to live by. Lack of flexibility in our lives can make our bones brittle. Bone deformities represent mental strains and pressures, or the state of being mentally stuck. If you have bone trouble, stop judging—accept yourself and others unconditionally. Trust the wisdom of Nature, and try to see the hidden meaning behind day-to-day happenings. A hunched back may represent lack of humility or accumulated anguish, and urges you to take responsibility and stop blaming others for this or anything else. Release all of your grudges.

The hips represent balance in life while stepping forward into the future. Rigidity in our attitudes, fear of the future and our ability to make and implement important decisions can all affect the flexibility of the hip joints. Providing Reiki at the hips may release many blocks and give you the peace and trust to make wise decisions in the future.

Arthritis

Arthritis—stiffness or pain in the joints—represents a conflict between the need to be approved by others as a nice person and the need to scold others for their apathetic behaviour towards us. The muscles near the joints get tired and stiff, obeying the conflicting unconscious commands of aggression and accommodation. Arthritic fingers, in particular, represent guilt and a desire to punish oneself.

Arthritic people may have confronted so many rejections and disapprovals while growing up that they judge themselves and others very critically, and go to extremes to be acceptable to others. They feel the safest situation is one where they are unable to *do* anything—and thus unable to make any mistakes. Immobile or arthritic joints create just such a situation.

In addition to judging and criticizing others harshly, especially people senior to them in either age or position, and blaming others for the imperfections in their lives, they tend to think there is only one way of doing things—as more than one way would require a decision, and present another opportunity to make the wrong one. Needless to say, arthritics find it hard to adapt to change, or to other ways of doing things; yet they hesitate to voice their preferences.

Recommended Affirmations: 7, 12, 16, 21, 25–26 and 28. Learn to love yourself and accept others unconditionally—start seeing love within, without and in-between. Forgive and release all your grudges and resentments against others, and watch arthritis begin to say goodbye.

Reiki Positions:

- Five minutes at each of the following: the affected joint, A4 and A5 together (for A5, keep the hand at the back of the head a little lower), B2–B3, B7, C3, C6, D1, across the shoulder blades and D5.
- Full-body Reiki with mental healing every other day, or whenever possible.
- For hip and leg pains: D1–D7 and the buttocks.
- For arm pains: D1, across the shoulder blades, and the top of the shoulders.

Dietary and Other Suggestions:

- Mix half a teaspoon of lemon juice and some honey in a

glass of water and drink it early every morning.

- Boil five teaspoons of dried gooseberries with almost double that amount of jaggery and a glass of water till it reduces to almost one third. Filter the mixture through a thin cloth and drink it twice daily.

- Adopt a vegetarian diet (including fish oil if you like, but not fresh fish itself). Eat plenty of whole-grain cereals, brewer's yeast, nuts, sweet potatoes, sunflower seeds, soybeans, tofu, bananas, avocados, mangoes, apricots, cantaloupe, oranges, broccoli, carrots, ginger, celery, Brussels sprouts, cabbage and other vegetables, especially green ones.

- Cut out refined foods, saturated fats, white sugar, white salt, tomatoes, eggs, eggplant, tobacco, white potatoes and peppers (except black pepper).

- Massage the affected area with hot mustard oil mixed with neem leaves, onion juice, salt and, if available, gourd juice.

- Garlic, gourd and sprouted fenugreek seeds are beneficial.

- Observe one-day fasts: eat nothing, and drink only carrot or cabbage juice. Repeat this fast on the 8th, 10th, 15th, 17th and 19th days of your regimen.

- Use canola (rapeseed) or olive oil for cooking. Minimise fried foods and margarines.

- Do Surya Namaskar for ten to fifteen minutes daily, followed by a session of yogasanas.

- Exercise: swim, play water games involving hand and leg movements against the water, cycle or walk regularly. Wear well cushioned shoes at all times.

- Relax through progressive relaxation, meditation or tai chi.

- Lose any excess weight.

- Train yourself to maintain proper posture (see suggestions under 'The Back', above).

Fractures

Fractures indicate a need to split from a particular aspect of our past, or to shift from a lifestyle of hectic materialistic physical pursuits to a more flexible, balanced, spiritual one. They can also indicate resentment and rebellion against superiors or seniors, or a weak or malfunctioning first chakra.

Recommended Affirmations: 7

Reiki Positions:

- Above and below the fracture (not *at* the fracture until the bone is set).
- After the bone is set, provide Reiki through the cast at the exact location of the fracture for at least fifteen minutes, at least twice a day. Follow this with both variations of A1, B3, C3, C6 and D7.

Dietary and Other Suggestions:

- Take a clove of garlic with each meal.
- Mix a pinch of turmeric into a tablespoon of honey and take it every three hours.
- Eat plenty of dairy products, nuts, leafy green vegetables and pulses (for calcium), plus oily fish (for vitamin D).
- Avoid bran, rhubarb, spinach and brown rice.

Osteomyelitis/Osteoporosis

Osteomyelitis is an inflammation of the bone or the bone marrow, usually due to infection. It reflects anger and disappointment at a life one finds unfavourable and inescapable, with nothing to fall back upon. Osteoporosis has similar causes—a feeling of lack of support in one's life. The bone marrow represents our core beliefs, and how we perceive ourselves, so all problems in this area represent low self-esteem or negative, defeatist or disempowering core beliefs.

Recommended Affirmations: 7, 16 and 22–25

Reiki Positions: A7, B2–B6 and D5

Dietary and Other Suggestions:

- Eat plenty of fish oil (salmon, sardine, tuna), spinach, wheat bran, brown rice, skimmed milk, cheese, tofu, nuts and rhubarb.
- Take plenty of milk and dairy products (especially children and adolescents).
- Cut down on smoking, alcohol, coffee, chocolate, salt, meat and bran (bran obstructs the absorption of calcium).
- Exposure to sunlight is valuable.

- Do yoga, tai chi, Surya Namaskar or Sudarshan Kriya.

Rickets

Rickets is the softening of the bones, especially in children, apparently because of a vitamin-D deficiency. Open yourself up to the sun's rays—the source of vitamin D—and to the energies of the universe, which come to us through feelings of stability, security and being loved and wanted by others.

Recommended Affirmations: 16, 22 and 25

Reiki Treatment: Full-body treatment, with or without absent healing.

Dietary and Other Suggestions:

- Get some appropriate, sensible exposure to sunlight every day, especially in winter and especially if your job keeps you indoors.
- Eat plenty of eggs and oily fish.
- Take vitamin D supplements under the guidance of a medical practitioner.

Scoliosis

Scoliosis is a side-to-side curvature of the spine. It afflicts more girls than boys, perhaps because it stems from a desire to be shorter than one actually is. Some children want to stay short so their elders will continue to find them 'cute', and the resulting unconscious tendency to 'curl within' manifests itself in a curvature of the spine. This desire is more pronounced in cases where a younger child has arrived in the family, usurping the attention to which the older child was accustomed.

Scoliosis can be treated if detected early enough in childhood. Appreciating tall children—especially girls who show early symptoms of scoliosis—can go a long way towards maintaining their upright spines.

Recommended Affirmations: 6 and 16

Reiki Positions: A6 and D1–D7. Reiki can benefit this ailment only if complete degeneration has not taken place.

Natural Supplements: Relax with yogasanas. The level of efficacy depends on how soon you begin treatment.

Sprains

Sprains result from unnecessary and forceful interventions in others' lives. Let others live the way they want to; voice your own feelings only if asked. If you must give unsolicited advice, give it only once, then step aside. Sprains may also represent resistance and anger towards the movement of one's life in a direction one does not prefer. Consult a physician to rule out the possibility of joint damage.

Recommended Affirmations: 4, 7, 9, 16 and 23–25

Reiki Positions: At least half an hour at the affected area. The pain may increase initially, but it will then subside. Follow this up with twenty minutes twice a day until the sprain is healed. Take care not to move the injured part during treatment.

Natural Supplements: Heat some powdered salt in a pan and place it between the folds of a clean, thick white cloth. Tie a knot around the salt to make a pack, and apply it warm to the sprained joint.

THE PALM AND FINGERS

The thumb represents the mind, so thumb injuries or problems represent worry. The index or Jupiter finger represents your ego or personality, so injuries here suggest a need to come to terms with your ego vis-à-vis a current episode in your life. (You may have fear, insecurity or anger relating to your acceptance by others.) The middle finger has to do with sex and anger. The ring or sun finger relates to sorrow or to running into someone you hate. The little or mercury finger pertains to family and to showing off.

Carpal Tunnel Syndrome / Cold Hands or Feet

Carpal Tunnel Syndrome occurs when a nerve in the wrist gets squeezed by swollen tissue. In one or both hands, the patient feels pain, numbness or 'pins and needles' in the wrist, thumb and index and middle fingers, making it difficult to hold objects. It is commonly associated with prolonged repetitive work such as typing.

Carpal Tunnel Syndrome, and the more basic problem of cold hands or feet, shows that you want something but feel you cannot get it or do not deserve it. You project anger and frustration on to the external world for what you perceive as its injustices. Numbness in the limbs indicates numbness of emotion, and a need to recognize those feelings one is avoiding or not bothering with.

Recommended Affirmations: 1, 3–4, 6–12, 14, 16, 21–25
Reiki Positions: Wrists, hands and all the positions listed under 'Arthritis', above.
Dietary and Other Suggestions:

- Eat plenty of yeast extract, wheat germ, oats, leafy green vegetables, bananas (all sources of vitamin B6) and the other sources of vitamins outlined under 'Neuralgia', below.
- Avoid smoking, alcohol, coffee, chocolate, tea and cola.
- Sit up straight, hold your arms at right angles and keep your wrists as straight as possible while typing. During long typing sessions, periodically raise your hands into the air and rotate your arm and wrists simultaneously for about two minutes.
- Do the exercises suggested under 'Stiff Neck', above, and 'Rigid Hands', below.

Rigid Hands

Lack of openness, bottled-up hostility and other negative emotions can manifest themselves in hands that stay clenched into a fist. Hands represent our potential to accept life's experiences, and the elbows represent our adaptability to change.

Recommended Affirmations: 7, 12, 16, 21, 25–26 and 28
Reiki Positions:

- Wrists, hands, and five minutes at each of the following: the affected joint, A4 and A5 together (for A5, keep the hand at the back of the head a little lower), B2–B3, B7, C3, C6, D1, across the shoulder blades, D5.
- Full-body Reiki with mental healing every other day, or whenever possible.

Dietary and Other Suggestions:

- Stretch your arms forward, parallel to each other. Let your hands hang limply, without any tension. Very slowly rotate your hands clockwise at the wrists. Exhale slowly, deeply and smoothly as you go up, and inhale the same way as you come down. Do this six times. Repeat by rotating the hands anti-clockwise. Do three complete cycles every morning and evening.

- To check your progress, inhale deeply and smoothly while clenching your fist, then exhale while opening it as far as it will go. With time, you will be able to open it farther and farther.
- Follow the suggestions under 'Arthritis', above.

THE LEGS AND FEET

Ankles

Our ankles reflect our ability to enjoy life. Guilt and rigidity keep us from doing so, and thus can cause ankle problems. Remind yourself that you deserve to enjoy life, and that happiness is nothing but a decision to be happy.
Recommended Affirmations: 2–9, 18–19 and 30
Reiki Positions: C2 and C5
Dietary and Other Suggestions:
Dry the seeds of a watermelon in a shady area. Pulverize them and pour two teaspoons into a cup of boiling water. Leave the cup undisturbed for an hour, then stir the liquid and pass it through a strainer. Drink it thrice a day to cure oedema of the ankles.

Corns

Corns are lumps of dead skin cells that result from constant friction and irritation between two adjacent bones and a shoe. Metaphysically, they are solidifications of accumulated pain.
Recommended Affirmations: 2, 6–8, 10, 16 and 22–25
Reiki Positions: C2 and C5
Dietary and Other Suggestions:
- Avoid the offending shoes in favour of more comfortable ones.

- Wash your feet regularly and use a pumice stone to remove rough skin.
- Every morning and evening, soak your feet in a bucket of hot water mixed with 125 grams of Epsom salts for ten minutes.
- Never attempt home surgery. It can have disastrous results, particularly if you are diabetic.
- Avoid wearing high heels.
- To relieve the pain, place good-quality natural wool between your toes.

Foot Problems

Feet show our understanding of ourselves and our lives. When you feel there is nowhere to go, it shows in your reluctant gait. Toe problems show minor but incessant worries about details of the future. Bunions show an inability to enjoy life. Like leg problems, foot problems ask us to change the pace at which we approach the future.

Athlete's foot, a fungal foot condition, indicates disappointment relating to disapproval by others, because of which one finds it difficult to flow with life. You must approve of yourself and trust in your destiny—with this kind of attitude, you will move towards the places and people necessary for your best interests at each point in your life.

Recommended Affirmations: 2–4, 6–9, 16, 22–25 and 34–35
Reiki Positions: C1-C7, elbows, palms over each other.
Dietary and Other Suggestions:

- Massage your soles with mustard oil every night before you go to bed. This aids in deep sleep, better eyesight, more energy and general podiatric health.
- To relieve hot or burning soles, rub gourd paste on them.
- Put your feet up.
- Soak your feet in a bucket of water mixed with two tablespoons of Epsom salts.
- Put your feet under tolerably hot running water, then switch to cold water.
- Wrap a sock filled with ice cubes around your feet and

ankles. Swab them dry with alcohol, cologne or vinegar.

- Avoid wearing high heels.
- From the ankle, rotate your big toe in a circle clockwise and then anti-clockwise, six times each. Do two complete sets. Point your toes down as far as they go, and then flex them up as far as they go, six times each. Do two complete sets.
- To get rid of foot odour, soak your feet for fifteen minutes twice a week in a quart of water mixed with half a cup of vinegar. Alternate shoes: do not wear the same pair of shoes on two consecutive days. Sprinkle some talcum powder within your shoes before putting them on. Wear only cotton socks, and change them twice a day if possible.
- For athlete's foot, mix one tablespoon of baking soda in a little lukewarm water and apply the paste to the afflicted spot. Rinse, dry and sprinkle talcum powder. Soak your feet in a bucket of water mixed with two tablespoons of Epsom salts. Keep your feet bare as often as possible; when you can't, wear only cotton socks, and change them twice a day if possible. Bind cotton wool dipped in honey or cider vinegar at the afflicted spot and leave it overnight. Drink two cups of fresh strawberry juice mixed with pulped fresh dates every day until the problem is cured.

Gout

Gout is a kind of arthritis involving inflammation of smaller joints (such as toes) due to excessive uric-acid salts in the bloodstream. It strikes all of a sudden, usually at night. The big toe is most often affected, but the knees, wrists and ankles may also get tender and swollen. Gout reflects anger, impatience and a need to dominate others—generally speaking, a rigid attitude towards everything. Nature uses gout to make you realise how stilted and impotent you make people feel with your anger, hostility and impatience. Relax, and learn to be kinder, more receptive and understanding of others.

Recommended Affirmations: 4, 7–8, 16 and 22–25
Reiki Positions: B6, across the shoulder blades, D5 and the afflicted areas.

Dietary and Other Suggestions:

- Drink ten to twelve glasses of water every day.
- Adopt a vegetarian diet rich in fresh fruits and vegetables (especially leafy greens), nuts, dairy products and fish oil (not fish or shellfish).
- Cut down on alcohol, dry beans and peas, asparagus, cauliflower, eggs, lentils and pulses, mushrooms, spinach, whole-grain breads and cereals, yeast, oatmeal and salt.
- Eat ¼ kilogram of cherries (look for plump and firm ones with green stalks to ensure their freshness) or drink their juice once a day if possible.
- Eat plenty of leeks, and drink tea brewed with celery seeds.
- Lose any excess weight. Do not attempt to fast, however, as it may exacerbate your gout.

Knee Problems

Stiffness in the knee joint may relate to rheumatoid or osteoarthritis. Often the problem is not in the knee but in the soft tissues around it—the muscles, ligaments and fascia that enable the leg to operate. Knee problems show our fear, inflexibility, arrogance, stubbornness, inability to forgive or tolerate ourselves or others and inability to adapt to change.

Recommended Affirmations: 2, 4, 6–9, 11–12, 16, 25 and 30

Reiki Positions: A1, C1, C3, C6, D1, and one hand on the sacral plate and other on the sole of one foot (repeat with other sole).

Dietary and Other Suggestions:

- Eat a cucumber with every meal.
- Grate a raw potato and apply it to the knee for fifteen minutes.
- Apply and release pressure with you thumb in the hollow at the outer sides of the knee located at four fingers breadth below the knee cap between the shin and the small bone.
- Lose any excess weight.
- Avoid any physical activity that puts strain on your knees.
- Find the point three inches above your kneecap and four inches into the inside of your thigh. Press this point with

your thumb and hold the pressure for a minute and a half. Relax, then repeat.

Do the following exercises regularly:

- Sit with your back against a wall, with a rolled towel tucked behind the small of your back. Roll a towel under your extended knees and try to tighten your muscles without moving the knees. Hold the tension for a count of six and then relax. Repeat twenty times. Now raise each leg six inches above the ground and hold for a count of six. Lower and relax for a count of six. Repeat twenty times. Do three sets.

- Lie on your stomach. With your knees slightly bent, raise one of your legs six to twelve inches above the floor and hold it up for a minute before bringing it very slowly back down. For better results, wrap a piece of cloth or a sock containing some coins or some other small weights around your ankles before you begin. Repeat six times.

- Lie on your back and fold your knees so your thighs are on your chest. Straighten your right knee and leg towards the ceiling and hold for five breaths. Repeat six times with each leg.

Legs

The legs represent moving ahead into the future. Fear or reluctance to move into the future may reflect itself in leg and foot problems, especially when we are not conscious of our fear. This often happens when we are oblivious of our life purpose. Look within—consider what you are good at, how you can serve others with these talents and what deep personal desires you have been overlooking. Once you discover your life purpose, you will realize the grand plan of the universe and feel freer to trust in your destiny.

Sciatica

Sciatica is intermittent but intense pain in the lower back, buttocks and backs of the thighs due to pressure on the sciatic nerve (which runs from the pelvis to the calf). Sciatica can also stem from a slipped disc or other spinal ailment, which in turn can be tracked down to malfunctioning of the first and/or second chakras. At the emotional level it represents hypocrisy, financial insecurity, fear of the future, fear of not being able to lead the kind of life you think you ought to and it asks you to check if you are trying too hard to prove yourself because of your low self-esteem. There is a great deal of unexpressed anger.

Slow down and relax. Trust that you are safe and secure wherever you go. The purpose of the universe is to ensure the greatest good for you always. When things do not go as we expect them to, we say they are going 'against' us—but Nature never does anything against us. His Holiness the Dalai Lama says that sometimes it is only by a stroke of luck that we do *not* get what we ask for. I have always believed that favourable luck is when we get what we want, but good luck is when we fail to get what we want, because those are the times when God's love is working to save us from some unknown misfortune.

Recommended Affirmations: 1, 6–7, 22–25 and 27
Reiki Positions: C4, C7, D7 and the elbow tips.

- Simultaneously at the sole of each foot and the area perpendicular to the spine, at the junction of the hips and lower back.
- For more elaborate treatment, place your hands horizontally across the tailbone and provide Reiki to the hip region; then move downwards, hand's breadth by hand's breadth, along the outer length of the leg to the arch of the foot. Spend about five minutes at each position. Repeat on the other leg.

Dietary and Other Suggestions:

- Give up alcohol, smoking and coffee.
- Grind a few castor-oil seeds and drink them with a glass of milk each morning.
- Take one teaspoon of garlic juice with some turmeric powder thrice a day.
- Boil some basil leaves and apply their vapours to the affected area using a handkerchief, at least once a day.

Varicose Veins

Varicose veins are those that get widened, distended and, in extreme cases, twisted when valves inside the veins (especially in the legs) break down, resulting in collections of excess blood. Symptoms include constant dull aches and pains and a general feeling of heaviness. Varicose veins express a feeling of being overburdened with work or responsibility without appreciation; and a general inability to enjoy our everyday work.

Recommended Affirmations: 2–4, 6–7, 9, 14, 16, 18–19, 21 and 25

Reiki Positions: B6–B7

Dietary and Other Suggestions:

- Stick to a high-fibre (starch) diet. Eat more whole-meal bread, brown rice, whole-wheat pasta, wheat germ, ginger, garlic, onions, black currants, citrus fruits, apples, pears, apricots, avocados, grapes and other fresh fruits, leafy green vegetables, seed oils and nuts.
- Drink ten to twelve glasses of water every day.
- Cut down on cakes and biscuits.
- Stop smoking.
- Do some regular exercise such as walking, swimming, cycling, yoga, tai chi or Surya Namaskar.
- If you have varicose veins already, avoid standing for long periods of time, and avoid crossing your legs while sitting.
- Lie down with your back on the floor and your legs leaning on a wall, pointing towards the ceiling. (Alternately, keep your thighs vertical but bend your knees over the seat of a chair.) Take slow, smooth, silent, deep breaths.
- Raise the head end of your bed four to six inches.
- Wear loose, comfortable clothing.
- Avoid constipation and obesity.

Weak and Tired Legs

Guilt and rigidity can also reduce the blood supply to the extremities, specifically causing trouble in the legs.

Recommended Affirmations: 3–4, 6–10, 16, 18–19, 22–23 and 25

***Reiki Positions*:**
- B2 and C4 simultaneously.
- B2 and C7 simultaneously.
- A1, D7 (T variation), C1–C3, C5–C6 and then one hand on the sacral plate and the other on the sole of one foot (repeat with the other sole).
- Place your hands crosswise on your thighs. Starting at the groin move downwards, hand's breadth by hand's breadth, towards the feet. Spend around five minutes at each position. Any pain that occurs is a positive sign.

***Dietary and Other Suggestions*:**
- Stop smoking. This is a must if you want relief. Do not read further if you are not prepared to do this; other remedies will not work if you continue to smoke.
- Adopt a wholesome vegetarian diet consisting of whole-grain cereals, seed oils, avocados, bread, pasta, and fresh fruits and vegetables.
- Give up alcohol. Cut down on salt, butter, cheese, full cream, tinned and smoked foods, brewed coffee, biscuits, potato chips, ice cream and chocolate.
- Drink plenty of water and other nourishing fluids such as soup and juice (not coffee, tea or cola).
- Eat one pineapple every day.
- Drink two tablespoons of wheat-grass juice thrice a day.
- Drink plenty of skimmed milk with a pinch of turmeric, garlic and onion each time.
- Lose any excess weight.
- Walk for an hour at least four days a week. Rest during your walk only if the pain gets moderately severe. If the weather does not permit walking, run in place, ride an exercise bike or climb stairs indoors.
- Do tai chi every day.
- Have a cardiologist check your blood pressure and cholesterol levels and look for blockages.
- Lie down with your back on the floor and your legs leaning on a wall, pointing towards the ceiling. (Alternately, keep your thighs vertical but bend your knees over the seat of a

chair.) Take slow, smooth, silent, deep breaths.

- Have someone massage your legs, from thighs to feet.
- Watch your posture. Do not cross your legs; keep your feet flat on the floor.

THE NERVOUS SYSTEM

Multiple Sclerosis

Multiple sclerosis is a chronic and progressive hardening of body tissue, resulting from damage to the sheaths around the nerve fibres in the central nervous system. The patient experiences numbness, fatigue and impairment of muscular coordination. Often MS develops when the patient is unable to see that he or she is trying to control everything around him or her. Multiple sclerosis is your body's attempt to make you realise that it's time to soften your mind and heart and let go of your fears, your rigid stance towards life and/or your need to control others. Make yourself more flexible: accept events and people as they are. Learn progressive relaxation, yoga nidra and/or meditation. Listen to the guidance that speaks into the calmness that ensues.

Recommended Affirmations: 3–4, 6–9, 12, 16, 18–19, 22–25 and 28

Reiki Positions: Full-body Reiki (preferably twice a day) with extra time on the afflicted areas; A1–A2 and A4–A5; both hands on top of the head and, if another practitioner is available, on the soles of the feet simultaneously; B3 and B5–B6; across the shoulder blades.

Finally, place both hands horizontally across the top of the spine (where it meets the skull) and move downwards, hand's breadth by hand's breadth, to the tailbone. Spend around five minutes at each position.

Dietary and Other Suggestions:

- Place more red and orange in your surroundings, wear red and orange more often and meditate on red and orange for ten minutes daily.
- Switch to a low-fat, high-fibre diet. Eat more whole grains, cooked leafy green vegetables such as spinach and kale,

carrots, red peppers, mangoes, cantaloupes and other fresh fruits. Cook with sunflower, safflower, corn or soya oil.

- Cut out white sugar, chocolate, pulses, beans, peas, lentils, white bread, pasta, peanuts and all salted nuts, spicy food, tea, coffee, cola, dairy products, meat, smoking and alcohol. You can drink weak lemon or herbal tea and decaffeinated coffee.
- Drink ten to twelve glasses of water every day.
- Do yogasanas and Sudarshan Kriya or, alternately, pranayama under the guidance of an experienced teacher.
- Have frequent massages.
- Lose any excess weight.

Nervous Breakdowns

The nerves are communication channels that tie us into a whole. Blocks in the nerves stem from a rigid, self-centered attitude and can result in nervous breakdowns—periods of mental illness marked by mental exhausion, fatigue, listlessness, depression and anxiety.

Recommended Affirmations: 7,12, 16 and 22–25

Reiki Positions: A1, A4, top of the head, B6–B7, C3, C6, D1, across the shoulders, and D7 (T variation).

Dietary and Other Suggestions:

- Take vitamin B capsules under the guidance of a physician.
- Drink lemon or rosemary herbal teas.
- Do yoga, pranayama (Sudarshan Kriya) or meditation.
- Have frequent massages.

Nervousness

Nervousness is an expression of inner disturbance, stress, fear, impatience, lack of peace, unnecessary haste, anxiety, and a disharmonious, undisciplined lifestyle. It is caused by brooding rather than acting; excessive thinking at the expensive of living and doing; and being pressured to perform.

Recommended Affirmations: 7, 12, 16, 17 and 22–25

Reiki Positions: Across the top of the head; A1 (on the sides of the nose), A2, A6, B2, B6, C3, C6, and the top of the foot.

Dietary and Other Suggestions:
- Have oatmeal for breakfast, and eat plenty of honey.
- Take plenty of the following through their natural sources (take supplements only on the advice of a physician): vitamin B complex (potatoes, preferably with skin, green vegetables, seeds, beans, pulses, brown rice, blueberries, betel nuts, brown bread), vitamin E (safflower oil, nuts, olive oil, avocados), vitamin C (gooseberries, citrus fruits).
- Eat more salads. One day a week, eat nothing but raw foods.
- Avoid tea, coffee and chocolate.
- Do half an hour of yogic exercise or ten to twelve minutes of tai chi each day.

Neuralgia

Neuralgia is an inflammation or compression of, or damage to, a nerve somewhere along its route. Shingles, sciatica, trigeminal neuralgia (involving nerves on the side of the face) and carpal tunnel syndrome (involving the wrists) are the main examples. Neuralgia has its roots in guilt over having failed to become 'complete' due to lack of effective interpersonal communication.
Recommended Affirmations: 2, 5–6, 26–27 and 30
Reiki Positions: Afflicted areas, A1–A6, C2–C3, C5–C6, and distance or mental healing to the whole being.
Dietary and Other Suggestions:
- For trigeminal neuralgia, apply pressure with the index fingers for seven or eight minutes every half hour at the inner end of the eyebrow on the affected side, and/or down towards the jaw, near the corners of the mouth.
- To relieve facial pain, apply a tablespoon of carrier lotion mixed with two drops of clove oil and one drop each of basil and eucalyptus oil.
- Take plenty of the following vitamins through their natural sources: vitamin B12 (whole-meal bread, brown rice, wheat germ, nuts, pulses, green vegetables), vitamin B1, also known as thiamine (potatoes, preferably with skin, brown rice, seeds, beans, blueberries, betel nuts, brown bread), vitamin E (safflower oil, nuts, olive oil and avocados) and vitamin C

(gooseberries, citrus fruits).
- Drink a weak infusion of rosemary.

Paralysis

Disease or injury to a muscle, or to the part of the nervous system that directs it, may result in the impairment or total cessation of motor functions. At a subconscious level, paralysis gives one the desired excuse to shirk one's responsibilities; it is often triggered by shocking news or extreme fear. Trust life, and learn to be open to all possibilities.

Recommended Affirmations: 4, 7, 16 and 22–25

Reiki Positions: Full-body Reiki twice daily, preferably with symbols. Spend extra time on A5, D5 and the afflicted areas.

Dietary and Other Suggestions:
- Take one onion with every meal.
- Drink one glass of bitter-gourd juice every day.
- Take honey in hot water.
- Mix some basil leaves, powdered rock salt and curd and rub on the affected area daily.
- Drink one or two glasses of mixed apple, grape and pear juice (in equal quantities) every day for a month.
- Take 25 grams skinned garlic and boil in milk till it gets almost pasty and viscous like gum. Cool it before eating. Take garlic, mustard oil and water in a 1:2:8 ratio and boil in an iron cauldron till no water is left. Cool it and massage the body of the patient with it. Carry on with this massage treatment for a month.

Parkinson's Disease

Parkinson's is a progressive disease of the nervous system resulting in tremors—involuntary movement of the muscles, especially those in the hands—plus muscular rigidity and the emaciation of resting muscles. Eventually the face wears a blank expression, with the mouth usually open, the speech choppy and saliva present in excess amounts. The patient tends to lean forward and walk slowly, with difficult, short jerky steps. The condition is also marked by loss of appetite, difficulty chewing and swallowing, weight loss and sluggish bowel movements. It is caused by degeneration of the ganglia group of nerve-cell bodies and a shortage of the neurotransmitter dopamine. Metaphysically, Parkinson's results from fear, which leads one to try to control everything and everyone.

Recommended Affirmations: 3, 7, 16, 18, 22–25

Reiki Positions: Full-body Reiki twice daily, with extra time on A1–A6, B3, D5 and both hands.

Dietary and Other Suggestions:

- Eat smaller meals more often.
- Drink ten to twelve glasses of water every day.
- Take proteins and unsaturated fats only in moderate amounts. Reduce your intake of saturated fats, tea, coffee and sugars, and increase that of fibrous foods—figs, prunes, papaya, pineapple, vegetables and whole grains.
- Do a visualization exercise: imagine that the neurotransmitter dopamine is being replenished in the brain.
- Do yogasanas and pranayama every morning.

Poliomyelitis

Poliomyelitis, or polio, is an infectious viral disease involving inflammation of the nerve cells in the spinal cord. It results in emaciation of the skeletal muscles and temporary or permanent paralysis leading to disability and/or deformity. Polio suggests that one is carrying jealousy to an extreme, and is in fact wishing that someone else would be paralysed.

Recommended Affirmations: 1, 7 , 9 and 21

Reiki Positions: Full-body Reiki, with extra time on the limbs.

Dietary and Other Suggestions:

- Do regular tai chi under the guidance of a practitioner who has experience with polio patients.
- Do regular yogasanas.
- Take up hydrotherapy, i.e., needle sprays or vortex baths followed by specific exercises in a hydrotherapy pool.

THE SKIN

Our skin is not only for sensing things but also represents our individuality: how secure we feel about ourselves, how we make contact with others, how we define the boundaries we set between ourselves and others and generally how we feel about ourselves. Skin problems manifest our anxieties about living up to our self-image and to others' perceptions of it, as well as problems relating to individuality—our ability to make contact with others or share tenderness with others. Sensitive people have sensitive skins, while thick-skinned people are indeed thick skinned. Acne affects mainly teenagers, but elderly people who dislike themselves are also vulnerable to a variety of skin diseases.

Abscess/Boils

An abscess is a tender, pus-filled inflammation in a body tissue, most commonly the gums. Physically, it is a natural response to a bacterial infection or other irritant. Metaphysically, an abscess draws your attention to an inner conflict you have been ignoring *or* have been obsessively preoccupied with—particularly thoughts of a hurt or slight that you wish you could avenge.

A boil is a type of abscess—in this case, a red, painful pus-filled inflammation that forms in the minute hollow around a hair follicle. Boils tend to erupt in hairy or friction-prone areas such as the nostrils, armpits, wrists, buttocks, or between the thighs. Pus consists of dead follicles and surrounding cells killed by a bacteria called staphylococcus. Boils usually erupt when one feels weak, run-down, tired or particularly diabetic. Though not usually serious, they should not be ignored: if the infection spreads, pus can enter the bloodstream and cause blood poisoning. For this reason, boils should never be squeezed, especially those that erupt near the lips, nose, armpit, groin or the breast of a nursing woman. When more than one follicle is involved, the cluster of boils is called a carbuncle.

Boils are a manifestation of suppressed 'boiling' anger. Get in touch with your innermost feelings by focusing your complete attention on your thoughts as you place your hands on your solar plexus. Continue observing your thoughts without being carried away with them.

Recommended Affirmations: 2, 7, 9 and 16
Reiki Positions:
■ For the tendency to lose one's temper: wrists, C3, C6, B3,

B6, D1, D7 and six inches above the ankles.

- For an abscess, treat the affected area directly: cover the abscess with a tissue, or channel Reiki from an inch above, for half an hour twice daily. Follow this with five to ten minutes on B5.

Dietary and Other Suggestions:

- Hold a thin, juicy slice of lemon, a soft-baked onion, some mashed garlic, the outer leaves of a cabbage, a bag of black tea or a heated slice of tomato on the abscess or boil with the help of a cloth or bandage.
- Apply a wet, warm compress to the affected area, changing it to retain warmth as often as necessary. Do this for about half an hour, three or four times a day. Continue for three weeks after the boil opens. Eat plenty of raw garlic and foods containing zinc and vitamins A, C and E (see 'Acne', below).
- Always keep your hands clean, and wash them with an antiseptic soap before eating or cooking.

Acne

Acne is a condition marked by unsightly spots on the face and sometimes on the chest, shoulders and back as well. Overproduction of sebum (oil), a substance produced to lubricate the skin and carry away dead skin cells, can block the sebaceous glands, resulting in clogged pores (blackheads) or red, sometimes pus-filled inflammations (pimples). Overproduction of sebum is caused by overproduction of the androgen hormones, which in turn is caused by foods that provide the body with excess iodine.

Acne is the physical surfacing of something you have been hiding out of shame or fear of disapproval: namely, in spite of your desire for intimacy with others, you resist intimacy at the subconscious level. You need to recognize and respect your deep need for closeness—do not let your ego interfere. You let your ego interfere with your longings because you lack love for yourself and in some way disapprove of yourself.

Acne usually strikes during puberty, though it can last into adulthood. Conflicts and guilt associated with growing up are common ingredients in the recipe of emotions resulting in skin problems. Teenagers often take their parents' objections and 'No's' as criticism or threats to their individuality. Low self-esteem only exacerbates skin problems. Unable to vent their grudges and anger, mostly against their parents, teenagers vent these feelings through pimples. In these cases parents cannot always help their children directly, as any suggestion from them is likely to be heard as criticism; but strengthening the patient's self-esteem may pave the way for easy recovery.

Recommended Affirmations: 26–27

Reiki Positions: Five minutes at the affected area and at A4–A6, B2–B3, B5–B7, D1 and D5–D7.

Dietary and Other Suggestions:

- Do not squeeze pimples.
- Wash your skin frequently to keep it free of excess oil. Avoid harsh, chemical-based soaps; rather, use mild, unscented varieties, ideally a medicated soap meant especially for acne.
- Eat a garlic clove with each meal, or rub it over the spots. Alternately, rub the spots with a little lemon juice.
- Vigorously rub your back, shoulders and chest with a dry towel once a day after bathing, to stimulate blood circulation to the skin.
- Women should avoid heavy or greasy makeup. Remove makeup every evening with a natural cleanser, then apply an oil-free moisturizer.
- Take two tablespoons of wheat-grass juice thrice a day.
- Drink a glass of warm water mixed with two teaspoons of honey thrice a day.
- Get plenty of vitamin A/beta carotene (carrots, apricots, mangoes, papayas, spinach) vitamin B complex (potatoes, preferably with skin, pulses, green vegetables, seeds, beans, brown rice, blueberries, betel nuts and brown bread), vitamin C (citrus fruits, gooseberries, black currants), vitamin E (whole-grain cereals, cold-pressed vegetable oils such as safflower oil, olive oil, nuts, eggs, avocados, sunflower seeds) and zinc (shellfish, nuts, poultry, lean meat). If you take a zinc supplement, take one that provides copper as well. Take

a 30-milligram supplement for two weeks.

- Adopt a wholesome vegetarian diet consisting of whole-grain cereals and salads made with fresh fruits and vegetables.
- Avoid fast food and all junk foods—burgers, chips, salty snacks, cheese, fatty meat, chocolate, sweets, cakes, soft drinks and white bread. Cut down on alcohol.
- Eat your vegetables raw or lightly cooked. Grill, steam or bake rather than roast or fry your food. Drink skimmed milk rather than full-cream milk.
- Do shankh prakshalan under the guidance of a yoga expert.
- Do Surya Namaskar at a fast pace.

Blisters

Blisters are small swellings revealing a collection of watery fluid under the outermost layer of the skin. They form as a result of friction (e.g. ill-fitting shoes), burns, sunburn, insects bites, chemicals or irritating substances. Blisters indicate a lack of emotional support from one's elders.

Recommended Affirmations: 4 and 7

Reiki Positions: Provide Reiki to the affected area. If the blister hurts, cup your hands above it, an inch away from the skin.

Dietary and Other Suggestions:

- Wear acrylic socks (available from sportswear shops) rather than cotton ones. Research has proven that they absorb more friction and generally protect the skin better.
- Sprinkle powder on your feet before putting on socks.
- For large, painful blisters: sterilize a needle in a flame until it glows red-hot. Let it cool, and use it to prick the blister. Take care only to prick; do not remove the broken skin, as this will expose the very raw skin beneath.
- Simmer some cabbage leaves in milk for a little while. Cool them down and hold them on the blister for ten to fifteen minutes.

Burns

First-, second- and third-degree burns cause redness, blisters, and destruction of the skin respectively. Third-degree burns usually damage the muscles beneath the skin as well.

Metaphysically, burns are meant to remind you of your burning desire to share love with someone. Alternately, you need to 'consume' your anger by giving it attention rather than letting it fester in your subconscious.

Recommended Affirmations: 7, 12, 16 and 22–25

Reiki Treatment: Provide Reiki to the affected area without touching the skin. The pain will initially increase; after it subsides, continue for ten more minutes. In case of excessive burns, opt for full-body treatment with extra time on A1, B1, B3, C3 , C6, D5 and D7.

Dietary and Other Suggestions:

- Always leave blisters intact. Cool them with tap water mixed with sugar and a pinch of turmeric (do not use ice-cold water or ice).
- Do not use turpentine oil or anything hot.
- Boil some tea in water and let it cool. Take a clean cloth, dip it in the tea and use it as a very lightly tied bandage for the burns. Change it every fifteen minutes.
- Make a paste of water and sesame seeds and apply it to the burns thrice a day.
- Avoid alcohol and cut down on tea and coffee.
- Drink plenty of water and fruit juice.
- Eat plenty of fresh fruit and vegetables, pulses, grains and foods containing zinc (shellfish, nuts, poultry, lean meat).
- If you take a zinc supplement, take one that provides copper as well. Take a 30-milligram supplement for two weeks.
- Avoid alcohol, and cut down on tea and coffee.

Cellulite

Cellulite is a condition wherein fat gathers in folds, wrinkles or bulges on the hips, inner thighs, buttocks, and sometimes upper arms or lower abdomen, creating lumpy, dimpled skin that resembles an orange peel. Women are particularly susceptible. Though not scientifically proven, it is believed that cellulite stems from a build-up of waste from refined or processed foods. Metaphysically, cellulite represents bottled-up anger and guilt.

Recommended Affirmations: 2, 7–8, 11–12, 25 and 30

Reiki Positions: B2–B6, C2, C5, D5 and the affected area.
Dietary and Other Suggestions:
- Drink ten to twelve glasses of water every day.
- Adopt a low-fat diet rich in fruits and vegetables and their juices. Drink plenty of beet-root, celery and cucumber juice, and eat plenty of watermelon.
- Take seaweed tablets and Spirulina capsules or tablets.
- Eat slowly and chew your food well.
- Cut out tea, coffee, alcohol and chocolate, and cut down on salt. Avoid ice-cold drinks.
- Have regular massages.
- Do some regular exercise such as swimming, walking, cycling, dancing, Surya Namaskar or yogasanas.
- Relax with progressive relaxation or yoga nidra, pranayama or Sudarshan Kriya.
- Lie with your legs propped up against a wall for ten minutes every day.

Cuts

Bleeding cuts show anger, disappointment and our frustration at not being able to meet our own expectations.
Recommended Affirmations: 7–8, 13, 17 and 21
Reiki Treatment: If you are bleeding, stem the flow or (if bleeding is heavy) seek immediate medical help. Before cleaning and bandaging, provide Reiki to the cut or wound itself (without touching it); continue till the bleeding stops. Provide Reiki regularly afterwards to ensure speedy healing.

If a great deal of blood is lost, provide Reiki to A1, A6, B5, C3, C6 and D5. For long-term preventive treatment, focus on A4, B1–B2, C3, C6 and D7 (both variations).
Dietary and Other Suggestions:
- Keep the wound covered with a breathable bandage.
- If the wound is large (more than a finger's width) or deep, call for medical assistance. Until it comes, wash with Dettol diluted with clean water. Place a clean cotton cloth, bandage or towel on the wound and apply direct pressure to stop the bleeding. If blood saturates the bandage, change it or add a

bandage or two on top. If bleeding does not stop, maintain the pressure and raise the affected area above the heart.

- Apply and maintain pressure on the pressure point closest to the cut, on the side towards the heart. Pressure points are points where you can feel your pulse: inside the wrists, halfway down your upper arm, and in the groin. Release the pressure a minute after the bleeding stops.

- Apply garlic paste to the wound as soon as possible.

Eczema

Eczema is a condition of inflamed, persistently itchy skin, often accompanied with weeping blisters and dry crusts and scabs. It is caused in large part by a food allergy. There are of two types of eczema: contact and atopic. The first can be caused by contact with irritants such as wool or synthetic clothes, certain metals, cosmetics, acrylic nail polish, detergents, sunlight, certain chemicals, raw fish, onions and garlic. Atopic eczema usually affects people who have a family history of asthma, hay fever or nettle rash. Symptoms for both varieties include redness, itching, dry, flaky skin and point-sized weeping blisters. Metaphysically, eczema stretches a barrier between you and others due to emotional threats, irritations, hurts, resistance and anger on your part. Become aware of your feelings, and accept things as they are.

Recommended Affirmations: 16 and 22–25

Reiki Positions: Full-body Reiki with extra time on A1, plus at least five minutes at A6, B1, B3–B4, B6–B7, D1–D2, D5 and the affected area.

Dietary and Other Suggestions:

- Make a note of what you eat and how, if at all, it affects your eczema. For two weeks, avoid all foods that may trigger or exacerbate the symptoms: milk, eggs, shellfish, wheat, tomatoes, apricots, nuts, soya products, yeast, chocolate, coffee, beer, tea, fatty foods and food with additives. If the eczema disappears, slowly start reintroducing these foods— one by one—into your diet and see if you can find the 'culprit'. Similarly, avoid touching things, edible or otherwise, that seem to trigger irritation.

- Wash, pound and warm some fresh, green cabbage leaves (especially savoy cabbage). Every morning and evening, hold several layers of them on the affected area with the help of a bandage for fifteen minutes.
- Make sure your laundry detergent is rinsed out thoroughly. Rinse twice if necessary.
- If you have eczema, avoid sudden changes in temperature—do not go from, say, an air-conditioned room into a steam bath. Wear cotton clothes; avoid synthetic fabrics.
- Use oatmeal powder tied in a handkerchief as your bath soap. Bathe in lukewarm (rather than hot) water. If you take a bath rather than a shower, put two tablespoons of sodium bicarbonate in your bathwater.
- Put some ice cubes in a glass of milk and let the milk chill for a few minutes. Filter the milk through a thin piece of cotton and apply the cotton to the affected area. Keep re-soaking and reapplying for ten to twelve minutes.
- Keep the affected area from dryness by applying almond, avocado or wheat-germ oil.

Growths/Nodules/Warts

Growths stem from resentments, from clinging to old hurts and slights. Nodules are small, rounded lumps of tumour tissue that indicate painful problems related to your career. Warts are small, hard, round, virus-induced projections composed mainly of enlarged skin cells. They are benign, but since they appear on the outer layer of skin, they are infectious. Warts mirror your guilt over some aspect of your life that you consider dirty.

Remember that the universe is beautiful and everyone in it, including you, is uniquely beautiful. Your imperfections have a purpose—they teach you to accept yourself and life as they are.
Recommended Affirmations: 1, 6-7, 9, 16, 21, 24–26 and 30
Reiki Treatment: If you are Reiki II or above, provide distance/intention Reiki in addition to the list below, visualizing your warts having been cured.

Channel Reiki daily to:

- The affected areas, B6 and the whole body until you see the signs of a healing reaction (aggravation of symptoms, darker urine, changed bowel movements, etc.). After that, channel for five minutes each at A1, A6, B1–B7, C3, C6, D5 and D7.
- The wart itself (pinch it lightly between the fingers) for ten to twelve minutes.

Dietary and Other Suggestions:

- Drink lots of water and juices to assist Reiki in the detoxification process.
- Leave warts alone—do not scratch them. If you are not sure how to identify a wart, see a doctor to make sure you don't have something more serious.
- Apply onion juice, a slice of raw potato or some coriander paste to the wart for fifteen minutes thrice a day.
- Apply castor oil (alone, or mixed into a paste with baking soda) to the wart directly twice a day.
- Apply a paste of ginger, garlic and honey directly to the wart twice a day.
- Soak some lemon slices in apple cider with a pinch of salt. Let the mixture sit for a fortnight, and then rub the slices over the wart.
- Rub your saliva on the wart soon after you get up in the morning.
- If you have plantar warts (plantar warts appear on the sole of the foot and grow within, rather than outward), tape the inside of a banana skin over them as often as possible.
- Eat a clove of garlic thrice a day.
- Take a capsule of 25,000 IU of natural vitamin A from fish oil, and rub its contents over the wart. Do *not* take it orally unless directed by a physician. Do this once daily until the wart disappears, which may take a few months. Alternately, rub the wart with the paste of a vitamin-C tablet pulverized in water. Be careful to restrict application to the wart itself.
- For five minutes twice a day, visualize your warts shrinking and dissolving.
- Use a self-hypnosis tape that suggests dissolution of warts.

(You may need to modify an existing self-hypnosis tape with your own voice for this purpose.)

Insect Bites

Insects detect with their feelers the weaker points along the acupuncture meridians, and attack them by injecting venom into the skin. The resulting pain, redness and swelling can last anywhere from a few hours to a full day. As with other accidents, insect bites are no coincidence—they represent your vulnerability to slights, insults, guilt and irritation over minor day-to-day happenings. Correspondingly, some people are more prone to these bites than others. Animal bites represent our anger towards ourselves, and our need to seek punishment.

Recommended Affirmations: 5 and 30

Reiki Positions: To prevent bug bites: five minutes at A1 (on the sides of the nose), B2 and B7. Once you have a bite: the affected area, without touching it.

Dietary and Other Suggestions:

- Remove the stinger if possible. Do not squeeze the stinger or the bite itself.
- Rub toothpaste, olive oil, lemon juice, alcohol, vinegar, baking-soda paste or garlic on the bite to relieve the itch.

Itching

Itching might be related to a skin disorder such as eczema, hives or scabies, or it might be related to excessive bile in the blood due to a liver disorder. Other causes are mosquito bites, dandruff, synthetic-fibre clothing, piles, worms, lice, anxiety and deep psychological problems. Itching reminds you of an unfulfilled desire or wish; it could be a wish to experience physical closeness with someone, or a need to acknowledge your bottled-up anger.

Recommended Affirmations: 7, 16 and 22–25

Reiki Positions: B3 and B5–B6. For itching caused by eczema and piles, see the sections on those ailments.

Lupus

Lupus is a disease of the immune system which turns the body's defense mechanism back on itself, leading to an ulcerous skin condition and sometimes damage to the connective tissues, joints and muscles, and major organs. Lupus starts with headaches, fatigue, muscle and joint pain and a rash on the cheeks and bridge of the nose. Patches appear on the skin, and new patches replace them as they heal, ultimately forming scales. Symptoms may also include lung infection and fever. Lupus is often triggered by exposure to sunlight, by certain drugs and by emotional upset. Metaphysically it indicates utter hopelessness, anger towards oneself and a desire to punish oneself.

Recommended Affirmations: 7, 10, 16, 22–23 and 25–29
Reiki Positions: Full-body Reiki with extra time at the afflicted areas.
Dietary and Other Suggestions:

- Avoid sunlight.
- Drink ten to twelve glasses of water every day.
- Take plenty of sardines and other oily fish (for omega-3 fatty acids), eggs, butter, milk and margarine (for vitamin D), low-fat dairy products (for calcium), apricots, broccoli, carrots, cabbage, cantaloupes, cauliflower, cabbage, and spinach (for beta carotene), citrus fruits, gooseberries and black currants (for vitamin C), and shellfish, oysters, nuts, poultry and lean meat (for zinc). If you take a zinc supplement, take one that provides copper as well. Take a 30-milligram supplement for two weeks.
- Give up alcohol and cut down on salt.
- Lose any excess weight.

Rashes

When insecurity leads you to ignore your emotions, they burst out physically in a rash. You may also be seeking attention from others, or be concerned over minor delays. Become more aware of your feelings, and stop seeking others' approval. Once you get your own approval, that of others will follow.

Recommended Affirmations: 18
Reiki Positions: Full-body treatment with extra time on A1, A6, B3, B7, across the shoulder blades, D5 and the afflicted area.
Dietary and Other Suggestions:

- Avoid mushrooms, grapes, wine, food with additives, and any form of yeast, mould or fungi such as bread, yeast extracts or cheese.
- Take plenty of leafy green vegetables, wheat germ and pulses.

Ringworm

Ringworm is a contagious fungal disease that erupts as ring-shaped discoloured patches on the skin. It erupts in moist, warm parts of the body such as the armpits, the groin (dhobi itch), beneath the breasts and between the toes (athlete's foot), though it may also involve the scalp, other hair follicles and the nails. Diabetics are prone to this condition when there is more sugar to feed the fungi. Ringworm reflects a strong disapproval or dislike of the self, particularly because one finds oneself worthless and dirty.
Recommended Affirmations: 7, 10 and 26–29.
Reiki Positions: A1, A6, B1, B3, B5–B7, C3, C6, D5, D7 and the affected areas.
Dietary and Other Suggestions:

- Cut down on alcohol, white bread, cakes, biscuits, sweets, refined sugars and starches
- Eat a clove of fresh garlic every day.
- Apply tea-tree oil to the affected spots.

Shingles

Shingles is a painful inflammation of the nerve ganglia, with a skin eruption often forming a 'girdle' on the middle of the body. It is caused by the same virus that causes chicken pox (herpes zoster), erupting when this virus, having lain dormant for years, gets reactivated. The reactivation of the virus may be triggered by stress or simply by contact with someone afflicted with chicken pox The first signs of shingles are severe pain and a burning sensation on one side of the body: the shoulder, waist, one side of the face, one eye, the chest, the back. The virus can be dangerous if it affects the eyes, as it can damage the cornea. These pains are followed by a rash, which may take two to three weeks to clear up. At the metaphysical level, shingles shows anger resulting from uncertainty and indecision. Trust the flow of life, and be open and receptive to the guidance God may be sending you. Believe that you will be guided throughout the journey that lies ahead, just as you have been guided so far.

Recommended Affirmations: 7, 16 and 22–25

Reiki Positions: Follow full-body treatment with a fifteen-minute application as follows: one hand on the left shoulder blade, the other at B1.

Dietary and Other Suggestions: On the appearance of the very first signs, start taking plenty of vitamin C and bioflavonoids (citrus fruits, apricots, gooseberries, black currants, cherries, tomatoes, papayas), vitamin B (whole grains, pulses) and vitamin E (sunflower seeds, avocados, whole-grain cereals, nuts, eggs, unsalted peanut butter, seed oils, olive oil and cold-pressed vegetable oils such as safflower oil).

THE URINARY TRACT

Bedwetting (Enuresis)

Bedwetting is natural enough in children less than four years old. Prolonged bedwetting, however, has a number of possible causes: anxiety, pressure to perform, psychological upset due to friction in the parents' relationship, a feeling of desertion due to a newly arrived brother or sister, urinary infection and difficulty learning to control the bladder.

As a parent, you must relieve the child of any psychological pressure you might be applying, and give him or her your unconditional love. Never try to stop bedwetting by frightening, warning or punishing the child—it simply does not work.

Recommended Affirmations: 13

Reiki Positions: For the child, A6, B6–B7, D1, D5 and D7. For the parents, provide intention Reiki with symbols to the correction of your attitude towards the child.

Dietary and Other Suggestions:

- Have the child drink lots of fluids during the day, and then practice bladder control by holding back urination as long as possible.
- Praise, encourage and reward the child for every dry night, and even more so for a pre-arranged goal of a certain number of dry nights. Some experts are of the opinion that the child should neither be praised nor scolded, as the child never does it on purpose, but this advice should be ignored. Change the sheet and let the child sleep on a dry area with a plastic or rubber sheet underneath.

Bladder Problems

Incontinence is far more common than most people think. Patients are often reluctant to speak of it for fear of embarrassment. Stress-related incontinence has the patient discharging a few drops of urine while coughing or straining or bending. A patient with urge-related incontinence feels the urge to urinate several times each hour, making it exhausting and potentially embarrassing for him or her to visit the toilet often enough. 'Dribbling' incontinence makes the patient urinate without his or her even knowing it. The bladder is never properly emptied, and the ceaseless urge continues.

Incontinence can also stem from a bladder infection, a stroke, a spinal injury, a bladder stone or blood cancer. Blood cancer can be caused by working too close to the chemicals used in dyes, and by excessive smoking.

A bladder infection (cystitis, caused by bacteria from the anus) manifests itself in burning pain during urination, plus abdominal and back pain. The patient urinates more often but only passes a few drops each time.

All bladder problems reflect long-standing psychological pressure or anxiety due to unexpressed disappointment, anger and resentment, especially (in women) towards the male partner. Incontinence is a physical 'escape' of bottled-up emotions. Talk things out with your spouse or a close, understanding friend, or simply write your feelings down. If you hold ideas or beliefs that seem worn out, replace them with newer, more relevant ones. Take a hard look at problems that press down on you, and try to resolve them.

Recommended Affirmations: 2–4 and 6–9

Reiki Positions: A4–A5, B6–B7, C2, C5, D1 and D7

Dietary and Other Suggestions:

- Empty your bladder as soon as you feel the urge. Don't wait.
- Eat a high-fibre diet.
- Drink plenty of cranberry juice.
- Lose any excess weight.
- Stop smoking. Cut out alcohol and coffee.

For cystitis:

- Use a hot-water bottle wrapped in a towel to relieve abdominal and back pain.
- To relieve the burning sensation, stir a teaspoon of bicarbonate of soda into a glass of water and drink it every three hours. (If you have heart trouble or high blood pressure, consult a physician before taking bicarbonate.)
- Avoid meat, vinegar, spicy food, tea, coffee, cola, cheese and citrus fruits.
- Drink a mixture of carrot and apple juice thrice a day.
- Eat plenty of horseradish and coriander seeds.
- Boil a tablespoon of barley in just enough water to cover it. Strain the barley and add some cold water. Simmer the barley with the rind of a lemon until it gets soft. Remove the barley and let it cool to lukewarm, add one or two tablespoons of honey and drink.
- Apply live yogurt to the skin above the affected area so its friendly bacteria can fight the germs.

Kidney Stones / Nephritis

The kidneys filter waste products from the blood into the urine, which in turn passes them through the bladder and out of the body. The kidneys also maintain balance among the body's fluids. Metaphysically, they mirror the state of our relationships with others. We often attract people (and partners) into our lives through whom we can live out an incomplete fragment of ourselves. You need to realize that the weaknesses and shortcomings you criticize so loudly in others are in fact projections of your own faults. Consider the kinds of problems you are having in relationships and what areas of life they lead you to work on. If you start recognizing these issues in yourself, you will not need to project them onto others.

Kidney stones hurt badly enough to bring tears to your eyes. The pain begins in short, severe bursts at the lower back, and travels down to the groin. Most kidney stones are calcium oxalates, usually formed when there is an infection, when the body is dehydrated, or when the density and concentration of stone-forming substances in the urine is high. Small numbers of solid particles are almost always present in the urine; the problem begins when the proportion of particles goes up and the urine is retained in the system. (High levels of stress can impede the flow of bodily fluids in the organs that carry them, such as the glands, ducts or bladder.) Extended stagnation of the urine allows particles to settle as a film at the bottom of the passage or organ, so when urine does flow over the film it thickens the accumulation of particles and eventually forms a stone. Peristaltic movements in the ureter tend to push the stones, resulting in pain and internal bleeding, both of which can spread to the abdomen and genitals (stones can even form in the uterus). Urination may become painful, and the urine may even carry blood.

Prolonged retention of your complaints and grudges, especially feelings of aggression towards your spouse or partner, can solidify in the form of kidney stones. Instead of focusing on what you have not got from your relationship, consider all that the relationship has given you.

Nephritis is an immune disorder in which antibodies attack the kidney's tissues, causing inflammation. The patient passes red or smoky-coloured urine in small quantities and suffers from headaches, backaches and high blood pressure. At the metaphysical level, nephritis indicates your extreme responses to life's failures and disappointments.

Recommended Affirmations: 2 and 17
Reiki Positions: A1, B6–B7, C2, C5, D5 and D7.
Dietary and Other Suggestions:

- Drink ten to twelve glasses of water each day.
- Urinate as soon as you feel the urge.
- Contrary to popular belief, continue with dairy products as more oxalates are absorbed in the absence of adequate calcium.
- Take plenty of wheat-grass juice, watercress, watermelon and well-washed leeks.
- Eat plenty of apricots, broccoli, pumpkin and cantaloupe or take vitamin-A supplements under a doctor's supervision.
- Cut down on animal fats, cheese, eggs and salt. Avoid low-salt substitutes, however.
- If you are susceptible to kidney stones, cut down on oxalate-rich foods such as beans, spinach, parsley, capsicum, rhubarb, beets, blueberries, celery, grapes, strawberries, chocolate, tea and peanuts. Also cut down on potassium-rich foods such as avocados, pears, bananas, pulses, seeds, dried fruits, coffee and powdered milk. (If you must eat potassium-rich fruit, stew and strain it first.)
- Do not take vitamin C or D supplements unless a doctor prescribes them or you are particularly susceptible to calcium stones.
- Avoid stress-inducing people and situations, and learn to be assertive about your needs. Aim to feel relaxed most of the time, perhaps by practicing yoga, yoga nidra, Surya Namaskar, meditation, or tai chi. Leave no stone unturned to ensure that no stones are formed!

Prostate Problems

The prostate is a walnut-sized gland that lies at the neck of a man's bladder and is involved in semen production. The urethra, the tube that carries urine from the bladder to the penis, passes through it. In men over fifty, enlargement of the prostate is a common problem; the inflammation can obstruct the flow of urine so that it comes in a thin, weak stream. The patient may feel frequent urges to urinate, particularly during the night, yet only pass a small amount of urine each time, and still feel that the bladder is not completely empty. Urination during the day may be difficult or painful. Metaphysically, prostate problems are often caused by misplaced evaluations and beliefs, pessimism, guilt, fear of getting older, fear of failing to achieve certain goals, a tendency to blame others for one's own faults or an inability to accept one's own masculinity .

Recommended Affirmations: 7, 21, 24, 27 and 30

Reiki Positions: At least ten minutes daily at A6, B2, B6, B7, D7 and under the perineum, and the area perpendicular to the spine, at the junction of the hips and lower back.

Dietary and Other Suggestions:

- Cut out meat, alcohol, tea, coffee and dairy products.
- Consume 30 grams of pumpkin and its seeds once a day.
- Eat foods rich in zinc, such as shellfish, lentils, chickpeas, nuts, poultry, lean meat, and/or take a 15-milligram zinc supplement daily.
- Eat foods rich in vitamin E, such as wheat-germ, safflower and olive oils, seeds, green vegetables, avocados, nuts and oily fish.
- Do yoga, tai chi, Surya Namaskar or another relaxation therapy.

Urinary Infections

Urinary infections represent deep dissatisfaction or annoyance at your spouse's or lover's behaviour.

Recommended Affirmations: 7–8, 11–12, 20–21 and 26–29

Reiki Positions: A4-A5, B6-B7, C2, C5, D1, D5 and D7.

Dietary and Other Suggestions:

- Drink plenty of fluids to flush out the offending bacteria. If your urine is not clear, you are not drinking enough water.
- Take a hot bath or shower.
- Eat plenty of coriander seeds, gooseberries, watercress and black currants.
- Always wipe yourself from back to front—not the other way around.

- Women prone to urinary infections should always urinate before and after sexual intercourse.
- Use sanitary napkins rather than tampons.

THE REPRODUCTIVE SYSTEM

Climacteric Problems

Fear of losing one's attractiveness and youth are often at the root of climacteric problems other than menopause.

Recommended Affirmations: 17 and 32

Reiki Positions: A5, B7 and D7 starting at least four days before the monthly period and continuing till the period is over.

Dietary and Other Suggestions:

Take calcium-magnesium supplements every other day for a month.

Dysmenorrhea

Dysmenorrhea is painful menstruation—that is, cramps in the lower abdomen and pain in the lower back or legs at the beginning of (or just before) a period. The cause is a tight cervix, which loosens up at the end of a pregnancy and brings the problem to an end. Symptoms usually last a day or two. Metaphysically, dysmenorrhea comes from looking down on your female body as a dirty and messy thing, feeling bad and unfortunate that you are a woman, and shying away from sharing your feelings with anyone else. Leaving such feelings unexpressed gives them no alternative but to express themselves through painful periods.

Recommended Affirmations: 6–7 and 14

Reiki Positions: A1–A3, A6, B3, B5–B7, C2–C7 and D5, D7 (T variation) and across the shoulder blades starting a week before the monthly period.

Dietary and Other Suggestions:

- Alternate hot (for two to three minutes) and cold (half a minute) compresses on the lower abdomen and back.
- Eat plenty of raw, fibre-rich fruits and vegetables such as mangoes, papayas, beans, carrots and lentils; citrus fruits

and gooseberries (for vitamin C); wheat germ, whole grains, brewer's yeast and leafy green vegetables (for vitamin B6); cold-pressed oils, sweet potatoes, and eggs (for vitamin E); and shellfish, nuts and dried fruits (for magnesium).

Endometriosis

Endometriosis is a condition wherein the mucous membrane lining the uterus begins to grow around the ovaries or Fallopian tubes, making it difficult to conceive a child. Small foci of this membrane may also appear in the intestinal cavity, interfering with the bowels and causing painful abdominal cramps.

Endometriosis comes from deep but unconscious feelings of deep dissatisfaction with being a woman. Often females grow up feeling that they are always at a disadvantage compared to males—they feel they are not as free as males, they need to work harder in the kitchen and around the house, they cannot stay outdoors late, they suffer the messy monthly business of menstruation and they must carry a child for nine long months when they get pregnant. However, some women take a different attitude towards their femininity—they feel that they have the unique ability to intuit, to see the 'big picture' and to be aware of their emotions. They take pride in pregnancy, birth and motherhood. They have a bond with their children that fathers cannot have. They feel that much of one's freedom has to be earned, and *can* therefore be earned with the right attitude.

Examine your feelings. If you feel disadvantaged because of your gender, acknowledge this consciously and perhaps share your thoughts with other women. Start seeing your femininity in a positive light—life is merely an interpretation. It never pays to have a negative interpretation of anything, especially when you cannot change it.

Recommended Affirmations: 17 and 32
Reiki Positions: A1–A3, A5–A6, B3, B5–B7, C2–C3, C5–C6, across the shoulder blades and D7 (T variation) and D5.
Dietary and Other Suggestions:

■ Press the pressure point at the junction of the thumb and index finger, and the tender one two inches above the ankle bone on the inside of the leg, five times for one minute each.

- Use sanitary napkins rather than tampons.
- If you need lubrication during intercourse, use egg white instead of commercially made jelly.
- Cut down on tea, coffee and all fizzy drinks.
- Do some moderate physical exercise such as walking, tai chi or yoga.
- For abdominal pain, apply a heating pad or hot-water bottle directly, or take some hot fluid such as soup. If heat does not help, try a cold pack instead.

Herpes

Herpes is a virus that causes blisters, fever and extreme discomfort—the infected area feels itchy and prickly. Blisters may appear on the genitals, lips, mouth, tongue, buttocks or near the eyes. The virus is usually picked up in childhood and remains dormant until reactivated by stress, exposure to excessive heat or cold, reduced resistance or, on occasion, menstruation. Herpes stems from a deep-seated sexual guilt or some kind of public shame, and a consequent need to punish oneself. This attitude is reinforced by a belief in God as an authority who punishes us for our sins, and a view of the genitals as instruments for 'dirty' acts.

Herpes simplex is a recurring form of herpes that afflicts the mouth or genitals. It stems from bottled-up bitter words that you have wanted to say but left unsaid. Remember that you alone are responsible for what happens to you, and it is only by forgiving and loving others that you can improve your life.

For herpes zoster, see 'Shingles', above.

Recommended Affirmations: 8, 12, 17–19, 32–33
Reiki Positions: The afflicted area and B6 for as long as possible.
Dietary and Other Suggestions:

- If you have blisters on your lips, apply a mixture of equal parts water and lemon juice thrice a day.
- Eat plenty of whole-meal cereals, wheat germ, brewer's yeast, fruits, vegetables, honey, milk and yoghurt. Cut down on sugar and refined foods.

- Eat plenty of carrots, apricots, mangoes, papaya and spinach (for beta carotene / vitamin A), potatoes (preferably with skin), pulses, seeds, beans, green vegetables, brown rice, blueberries, betel nuts and brown bread (for vitamin B complex), whole-grain cereals, cold-pressed vegetables oils such as safflower oil, olive oil, nuts, eggs, avocados and sunflower seeds (for vitamin E), citrus fruits, gooseberries and black currants (for vitamin C) and shellfish, poultry, nuts and lean meat (for zinc). If you take a zinc supplement, take one that has copper as well. Take 30-milligram supplements for two weeks.
- Wear cotton undergarments. Do not let woollens touch your skin.
- Do not touch the blisters—they are easily spread to other parts of the body.
- Take a bath with warm water. Do not share your towel.
- If you or your partner has herpes, do not have intercourse without a condom.
- Change your toothbrush after you find a cold sore in your mouth, and change it again after the sores heal. Store your toothbrush in a dry area, not in the bathroom.
- Get enough sleep.
- To strengthen your immune system, fold a flannel cloth in half and soak it in a little castor oil. Place it over your abdomen, cover it with a plastic sheet, place a heating pad or hot-water bottle over it and hold it for an hour or so. Between herpes attacks, do this once a day for a month, then every other day. During a herpes attack, do it several times a day.
- Do yoga, Sudarshan Kriya or yoga nidra.

Infertility

Infertility is difficulty conceiving a baby. Being stressed and worrying too much can make conception difficult, but on a metaphysical level infertility stems from a deep, unacknowledged reluctance or unpreparedness to take on the responsibility of parenthood. Sterility shows a deep fear of a close relationship and of taking parental responsibility. Nine out of ten couples manage to conceive a child within a year's time.

Recommended Affirmations: 13 and 24

Reiki Positions: A1–A6, B1, B6–B7 and D7

Suggestions:

- If you need lubrication during intercourse, use egg white instead of commercially made jelly.

- A woman is most fertile two to three days before and after ovulation. (The body temperature just before a woman gets up in the morning is higher by .2 to .5 degrees Centigrade when ovulation takes place.) Alternately, make love every night from day 11 to day 16 of the menstrual cycle after having abstained for two or three days (to enhance the man's fertility). Use the missionary position. The woman should keep lying on her back for twenty minutes after intercourse.

- A woman having trouble conceiving should avoid strenuous exercise in favour of lighter routines such as tai chi or yoga. Women who diet should dispense with weight worries for the time being, as abundant vital nutrients are essential for conception. Fat should constitute eighteen per cent of a woman's body weight; any less than that might interfere with ovulation.

- The man should keep his testicles cool by splashing cold water on them several times a day and avoiding bathtubs, extreme temperatures, excessive physical activity and tight underwear.

Dietary Suggestions: Three to six months before the planned conception, both partners need to give up smoking and drinking; get lots of vitamin C (citrus fruits, gooseberries) and zinc (shellfish, lentils, chickpeas, nuts, poultry, lean meat); and cut down on coffee, chocolate, cola and highly refined foods such as white flour and white sugar.

- Men should get plenty of vitamin A, vitamin B complex and vitamin E (see food suggestions in 'Herpes', above) and selenium, found in whole-grain cereals, fish, shellfish and brewer's yeast.

- To help oestrogen metabolism, women should get plenty of

vitamin B6 (whole grains, wheat germ, yeast extracts, green vegetables, oats, bananas, pulses, dried figs, sunflower seeds) and manganese (oats, wheat germ, chestnuts, rye bread, peas). Women should also get plenty of iron (red meat, fish, poultry, beans, lentils, whole-meal flour, oatmeal, nuts, parsley, egg yolk, fruits, dark-green leafy vegetables), folate (leafy green vegetables, beans, eggs, fruits, peanuts, yeast extract, whole-grain cereals), and magnesium (garlic, wheat-grass juice, whole-grain cereals, dried figs, nuts, pulses, parsley and leafy green vegetables).

- A woman's daily requirement of polyunsaturated fatty acids is 4 grams of the Omega 6 variety (two teaspoons of sunflower oil or a handful of almonds or walnuts) and 2 grams of the Omega 3 variety (two teaspoons of rapeseed oil or a handful of walnuts). Other foods with these fatty acids are soya beans, fish oil, other vegetable oils such as olive oil, and oily fish such as sardines, mackerel and salmon.

Menopause / Premenstrual Syndrome

The ovaries symbolize creativity. Menopause is the permanent stoppage of ovulation, and thus of a woman's monthly periods. Generally speaking, the word also refers to the symptoms that accompany this phase of waning fertility. Menopause usually begins in a woman's forties or mid- fifties, lasts two or three years and is somewhat upsetting both physically and emotionally. Symptoms such as hot flashes, night sweats, erratic extreme moods and depression mirror the underlying fear that age may reduce one's female attractiveness and ability to evoke desire in a partner.

Premenstrual Syndrome (PMS) refers to the physiological and psychological changes caused by the hormonal changes taking place just before menstruation. Symptoms can include fatigue, headaches, sore breasts, acne, inability to concentrate, irritability and depression. Metaphysically, PMS reflects three problems: you are not resolving the confusion in your life, you are letting others run your life for you, and you are not accepting your femininity or the processes involved with it.

Recommended Affirmations: 16-17 and 32
Reiki Positions: A4–A5, A1 (on the sides of the nose), B1–B3, B5–B7, D5 and D7.
Dietary and Other Suggestions:

- Get adequate sleep and regular exercise.
- Eat a balanced wholesome diet that is high in carbohydrates but low in fat. Eat plenty of oats, whole-meal bread, whole grains, wheat germ, red meat, oranges, gooseberries, olive oil, shellfish, oily fish, dried fruits, nuts, spinach and other leafy green vegetables, eggs and low-fat dairy products
- Work oats, soybeans and alfalfa sprouts into your breakfast.
- Eat smaller meals more often.
- Lose any excess weight.
- Cut out alcohol, and cut down on tea, coffee and salt.
- Wear natural fibres.
- Drink lots of water.
- Practise yoga, yoga nidra, Sudarshan Kriya, tai chi or Surya Namaskar.

Menorrhagia

Menorrhagia, or profuse menstrual bleeding, can be caused by a hormone imbalance or by fibroids or infection in the womb or Fallopian tubes. It occurs when we let our uterus weep instead of our eyes. Ask yourself what it is that you are not venting through your tears—what do you dread happening in the future? What upsets you right now?
Recommended Affirmations: 17 and 32
Reiki Positions: B3, B6–B7, C2–C3, C5–C6, D7 (T variation) and across the shoulder blades.
Dietary and Other Suggestions: Eat plenty of whole-meal bread, leafy dark-green vegetables, dried fruits and citrus fruit juices.

Miscarriage

Miscarriages are more common than you might think. In fact, only one fourth of conceptions result in live births. Miscarriages reflect a conscious or unconscious procrastination—a slight disinclination to welcome the child owing to tension and disturbance at home, fear of becoming a mother or any other similar problem. Similarly, a premature birth indicates the mother's impatience to deliver the child. Providing the unborn child with love, patience and Reiki will ensure that you do not deliver prematurely. Delayed births reflect the mother's inability to let the child go.

Recommended Affirmations: 3–4, 6–7, 9, 13 and 22

Reiki Positions: A2, B1–B3, B5–B7, C3, C6, D5–D7 and at the two outer junctions of hip and thigh. During labour, give hands-on or absentee group healing to the mother and unborn child at the above positions.

Dietary and Other Suggestions:

- The first three months of pregnancy demand a high-quality, high-calorie diet. Eat plenty of whole-meal bread, pasta, apricots, carrots, red peppers and other fruits and vegetables, dairy products, meat, eggs, pulses, nuts, seeds, seed oils and oily fish. Meat, poultry and eggs should be cooked properly to kill bacteria.
- Drink ten to twelve glasses of water each day.
- Throughout pregnancy, keep protein and salt intake at normal levels. Take one or more of the following each day:
  - Two oranges or a glass of orange juice.
  - A fresh coconut and its water.
  - Fifty grams of peanuts.
  - An apple, some carrots or some lemon juice.
  - Two teaspoons of honey or wheat-grass juice.
  - Zinc-rich foods such as shellfish, nuts, poultry and lean meat.

Sexual Problems

Sexual guilt and shame often result in genital problems. Many people grow up believing that sex is sinful or bad, and they feel guilty enjoying their bodies. Frigidity can stem from these beliefs, or from the fear that results. Impotence stems from pressure to perform well sexually, negative feelings about sex and the genitals, guilt, domination by an over-strict mother or emotional pain caused by a previous partner.

Most of these problems can be overcome if you start accepting your genitals as no less pure, sacred and beautiful than any other part of your body. Shed sexual guilt: forgive yourself, let yourself go and be willing to give and share love by trusting and believing in your sexuality.

Recommended Affirmations: 17 and 32-33

Reiki Positions: A1 (on the sides of the nose), one hand at B2 and the other at B7 (left, then right), D5, D7 and the perineum between the legs. In case of frigidity or impotence, provide *both* partners with full body Reiki with extra time on A5, A7, across the shoulders, B1, B6–B7, D5 and D7.

Dietary and Other Suggestions: Each day, drink a tablespoon of wheat-grass juice, eat some wheat sprouts and eat four or five cloves of garlic before drinking a glass of milk.

Vaginitis

Vaginitis, or inflammation of the vagina, is your vagina speaking the truth that you are hiding from yourself regarding your unhappiness about your relationship with your spouse or partner. Vaginitis shows sexual guilt, desire to punish oneself or our anger at our spouse or lover.

Recommended Affirmations: 7, 17, 26–28 and 32

Reiki Positions: Elbows, D1, D5, perineum and D7.

Dietary and Other Suggestions: Apply salt washes and live yoghurt to the affected area.

Venereal Disease

Venereal diseases show a deep but subconscious guilt relating to sex, and a perception of the genitals as negative and impure. Obviously, it is not sex but one's skewed attitude towards it that needs treatment. Sex is an expression of love, and of one's desire to share that love.

Recommended Affirmations: 17 and 32–33

Reiki Positions: To supplement medical treatment, provide Reiki to D7, B6 and A1.

Dietary and Other Suggestions:
- Cut down on coffee, tea and cola.
- Eat plenty of whole grains, fresh fruits and vegetables and their juices, and moderate amounts of lean meat, poultry, fish, nuts and pulses.

- Get adequate rest.

ADDICTIONS

Addiction is dependence on a substance or form of escape that alters the body chemistry or mood. One can be addicted to alcohol, drugs, smoking, tranquillizers, tea, coffee, chocolate, sex, pornography or just about anything else. As the body gets accustomed to the addiction, greater and greater doses are required to maintain the same level of stimulation. After a point, giving up an addiction becomes difficult—the patient may suffer headaches, stomach aches, anxiety, loss of appetite, insomnia, muscle cramps, nausea, vomiting, palpitations, sweating and even convulsions and hallucinations in the process of trying to quit.

Addictions indicate a desire to grow without working for it, an assumption that you can depend on something external for internal fulfillment. They also indicate a basic running away from life. If you feel the need to escape through alcohol or frequent sex (especially sex that stems from stress rather than love), you are clearly not enjoying life and are trying to fill the void. Alcoholism only aggravates the conflict, guilt or inferiority complex you are running away from. Ask yourself what it is that you are running from, what you do not want to face. You cannot make your problems smaller, but you can make yourself bigger than they are.

Recommended Affirmations: 15, 26–27
Reiki Positions: A1, A4, A6, B3, B5–B7, D1, D5–D7 and across the shoulder blades. For detoxification: mental full-body treatment.

Dietary and Other Suggestions:
- Make sure your diet is balanced and has all the necessary vitamins and minerals, especially vitamins B (B1, B6, B1) and C.
- For detoxification, see 'Reiki and Diet' in Chapter 3.
- Optional: do Surya Namaskar, yoga, yoga nidra, meditation or Sudarshan Kriya.

Overeating/Bulimia

Obesity usually stems from an undisciplined lifestyle with little physical activity and indiscriminate consumption of fatty and sugary foods. A diet that is high in fat and low in carbohydrates is likely to make you fat. Fat should not constitute more than thirty-five per cent of your total caloric intake. You are overweight if you are at least thirty per cent heavier than the medically acceptable weight for your height, sex and age. Apart from being embarrassing, obesity can threaten the health of your heart, pancreas, gall bladder and joints, and may result in shortness of breath, swollen ankles and aching legs.

Low self-esteem makes us more vulnerable to insults, criticism, abuse and pain and makes us throw around ourselves a protective shield or covering of fat. Many overweight people have a lot of accumulated fears, stemming from deep-seated anger and an inability to forgive themselves and others. Such people also feel a void or an uncomfortable emptiness in their lives, and want to fill it or escape from it with food. Obese people (especially children) who are particularly drawn to sweet things feel a lack of love in their lives. Fat accumulated at different parts of the body represents anger at different things. On the thighs, it represents anger accumulated during childhood, most likely towards the father. At the hips, it represents anger towards the parents; at the belly, it means one feels one was denied nourishment. On the arms, it represents anger at having been denied love.

If you are obese: before addressing your diet you must address your feelings of insecurity, and ask yourself what you are afraid of, what you are trying to protect yourself from. Love and approve of yourself, abstain from self-defeating negative thoughts and watch your body transform itself into an attractive and slender one.

Bulimia patients, or those engaged in cyclical overeating and vomiting, are often not even overweight. Bulimia nervosa is a stress-related eating disorder to which females are particularly prone. Many girls and women are over-concerned with being slim and shapely, and they adopt drastic crash diets that make them (naturally enough) crave food. To satisfy their cravings, they overeat, but to stick to their diets they induce vomiting (or take a laxative) afterwards—resulting in a vicious cycle of starving, binging and vomiting. Physical symptoms include swollen neck glands, irregular menstrual periods, swollen feet and ankles, irregular heartbeats and poorly functioning kidneys. Emotional symptoms are guilt, depression and, sometimes, a tendency to drink.

Recommended Affirmations: Tell yourself several times each day, 'I am getting lighter and thinner every single day.'

Once a day, hold a mirror in your hand. Looking at your face, smile and say:

- 'I love and respect myself immensely.'
- 'I accept and approve of myself completely. I am working towards a new personal reality.'
- 'I am proud of what I am, regardless of what others may think. What is important is how *I* feel about myself.'
- 'I am completely safe and secure. I know I am always looked after by the higher forces of the universe.'
- 'I am at peace with myself. I am already perfect, and happy the way I am.'
- 'I know my life is beautifully destined. Worrying cannot change it for the better. The trust and gratitude I have introduced into my life will improve it even further.'
- 'I take full responsibility for myself. I am what I have made myself with my thoughts. Since I have made myself what I am today, I can make myself the way I would like to be tomorrow.'

Recommended Attitudinal Changes:

- Respect yourself. Never say a negative word about yourself. If you hear negative words from others, refuse to accept them; just draw the appropriate lessons from them (if any) and move on.
- Do not be impatient for results. Trust in your path to a slimmer you, the course of which only Reiki knows.
- Visualize yourself being thinner.
- Live with an attitude of gratitude.

Reiki Positions: A2, A5–A6, A1 (on the sides of the nose), B2–B3, B5–B7, C2–C3 and C5–C6, D7 and across the shoulder blades.

Dietary and Other Suggestions:

For obesity:

- Drink ten to twelve glasses of water each day.
- For breakfast, eat only fruits and vegetables with a little salt.
- Eat slowly and chew your food well.
- Adopt a diet low in fats but rich in complex carbohydrates (pasta, potatoes, brown rice, whole-meal bread, fresh fruits and vegetables, and pulses). Drink plenty of fruit and vegetable juices.
- Avoid biscuits, cakes and full-fat dairy products.
- Cut out proteins (eggs, milk, meat, pulses), except a little curd.
- Cut out smoking and alcohol.
- Engage in some sport or physical activity that you enjoy,
- Do some regular exercise such as yoga, Surya Namaskar, tai chi, or pranayam such as Sudarshan Kriya.
- Meditate for twenty minutes daily.
- Do shankh prakshalan (a yogic kriya that cleans the digestive tract) under the guidance of an expert.

For bulimia:

- Gradually introduce a balanced, fibre-rich diet consisting of fruit and vegetable juices and foods rich in potassium (see 'Smoking', below).
- Cut out tea, coffee, alcohol, cola, chocolates and fatty foods in general.
- Avoid laxatives.
- Do not snack between meals.
- Set goals at the beginning of each day.

Pornography

Addiction to pornography is a sign of boredom, stress, repressed sexual desire, a wish to escape from difficult or uninteresting responsibilities, or simply a lack of joy in one's life. Often providing Reiki increases the craving initially, as it lets loose all that you have been repressing. Carry on with Reiki in the second and third chakras (along with the positions given below), always with an attentive mind. Be aware of your thoughts as you receive Reiki; unwind and let go of all your repressed 'trash'. Watch the lustful thoughts cross your mind without leaving any residue or footprints, just as birds leave no footprints in the sky. Observe them as if they are not yours but someone else's. In the future, whenever you become aware of such thoughts, do not get carried away with them; simply watch them with careful but indifferent attention. When the desire to see pornography arises, take a few slow, deep breaths and think or say the following affirmations:

'Pornography is only a mirage. It always promised to satisfy, but it never did and it never will.'

'I have come out of prison into the open sky, to breathe in and enjoy "real" life. I thank myself and God for that.'

'My need to watch pornography has been dissolved from within. I see this habit as a thing of the distant past.'

'I have learnt to shift my focus from a "great body" to be exploited for sensual gratification to a "lovable person" who is an expression of God's love and hence sacred.'

'It is simple—I am postponing it. I am not doing it now. Instead, I am breathing deeply and doing some physical exercise, or I am going out to meet some others.'

Stay away from people, places and situations that encourage thoughts of pornography. Keep yourself busy with others things, and stay in the company of family members or others with whom you cannot indulge this addiction.

Pray with deep feelings first thing in the morning, before getting out of bed: 'I resolve that, just for today, I choose to be without it. I *will* be without it. I know it is easy for me to do so. God, bless me with your infinite power to enable me to honour my resolve.'

Recommended Affirmations: See above.

Reiki Positions: A1, A4, A6, B3, B6, D1, D5 and across the shoulder blades.

Dietary and Other Suggestions:

- Meditate on the colour yellow for ten to fifteen minutes, either by imagining it or by looking at it directly.

- Locate the pressure point between the heel and the arch of the foot, towards the inner edge. Massage it gently, with steady pressure.

- Imagine yourself floating in water at night, looking up at the full moon. Feel how its light soothes your body. Imagine all your tension, negativity and lust being washed into the water.

Smoking

Two million people worldwide die every year because of smoking. You can quit smoking; it is never too late. If the habit is only ten to fifteen years old, quitting reduces your risk of heart disease to that of a lifelong non-smoker. You need not worry about gaining extra weight once you quit; you'll just have to reduce your fat intake and increase that of starchy foods such as pasta and potatoes. When you do quit smoking, take care not to replace the habit with another unhealthy addiction (such as chewing betel leaves or tobacco-based products), and to control any cravings for sweets, soft drinks and snacks.

Recommended affirmations: 15 and 26–27

Reiki Positions: A1, A4–A6, B3, B6–B7, C3, C6, D5 and D7. Give intention Reiki through symbols to the idea of yourself as a nonsmoker.

Dietary and Other Suggestions:

To starve the habit physically:

- First, give up smoking at or after meals.
- Then, cut out odd puffs every now and then.
- When you feel the urge, place a few drops of clove oil on your tongue. Taking chlonodine tablets and practising deep breathing can also help.
- Divert your attention from the urge by doing some work—make a phone call, go shopping, etc.
- Ask your friends to help you by not offering you cigarettes.
- Brush your teeth thrice a day.

- Eat more fruits and vegetables. Get plenty of potassium (nuts, dried fruits, pulses, whole grains, avocados, tomatoes, potatoes, bananas and oranges) and magnesium (whole-grain cereals, dried figs, nuts, pulses, garlic, wheat-grass juice, parsley and leafy green vegetables). Cut down on proteins, especially animal proteins including eggs. Milk and yoghurt can be continued in moderation.
- Avoid tea, coffee, alcohol, cola, chocolate and red meat.
- Take vitamin A, B-complex, C, E and zinc supplements.
- When you succeed, reward yourself with something you like—buy yourself a gift or spend some time and money on a favourite hobby, a movie or a game. If you fail, try again!

To *study the habit mentally*:

- Recognize the pattern by recording in your diary—when, where, why, the situation and the intensity of the urge.
- Remind yourself of the millions of others who have given up smoking. If they could do it, why can't you?
- Focus your attention on not smoking each individual cigarette, not on making a lifelong commitment.
- Remind yourself, one by one, of all the reasons to quit. Jot down the health risks, and imagine a life afflicted and cut short by lung cancer or heart disease. Think of the money you'll save.
- Choose the date and write it into your calendar. Disclose it to your friends and family members and look forward to it eagerly. The date should not be too far away, and should not be a day when you are likely to feel stress: changing jobs, appearing for an important interview or a court case, etc. A holiday can be a good choice.
- Tell yourself that it is getting easier and you are getting better with every passing day. Eventually, you will not need to make an effort to curb the urge.

To *replace the habit spiritually*:

- Do regular physical exercise.
- Meditate every day.
- Visualize your body as a spiritual shrine. This will help you see the need to keep it clean.

- Reduce your dependence on how others perceive you. Be yourself, and tell yourself that your only desire is to fit yourself into the larger cosmic plan by answering your inner spiritual calls.
- Rather than try to escape your worries by smoking, remind yourself that everything in life is temporary, including whatever you are worried about.
- Consult a hypnotherapist.

CANCER

Cancer refers to various kinds of malignant growths and the illnesses that result from them. Unlike normal body cells, cancer cells grow and proliferate rapidly and erratically, and have no useful role in the body's functioning. These cells invade, destroy and gobble up neighbouring cells at random, often spreading to distant areas through the blood stream and lymph cells and causing secondary tumours elsewhere. Cancer cells contain impaired genetic material that 'exempts' them from the body's homeostatic control, or state of equilibrium. External causes can include radiation, viral infection, hormonal imbalance, heredity, chemicals, stress and improper diet.

At the metaphysical level, cancer is the result of accumulated resentment, self-pity, grief or depression, disappointment, hopelessness, helplessness or lack of life purpose. People who find it hard to trust others and to maintain lasting relationships are prone to attract cancer. They tend to blame others and feel disgusted with themselves. Along with Reiki, developing high self-esteem may accelerate the healing process, especially if the cancer is in an early stage. Find out which facet of your life seems difficult to integrate with the wholeness of your being.

Warning signs: Below are some physical symptoms that *may* indicate the possibility of cancer. They are by no means definitive; they can, of course, indicate far less serious ailments. If they last more than two weeks, see a physician to rule out the possibility of cancer. Most cancers are now curable *if* they are detected early.

- Loss of weight or appetite, persistent fatigue, indigestion without obvious cause.
- A lump in the neck, difficulty swallowing, persistent cough (with or without blood), hoarseness.
- Blood in the urine or faeces.
- Change in frequency of bowel movements or urination.
- Change in the shape and size of a wart or mole.
- A wound that refuses to heal.
- Vaginal bleeding between periods, after intercourse or after menopause.
- Pain, itching, burning, a growth or boils in the vaginal area.
- Bloody discharge from the nipples.
- A lump or knot-like formation in the breast.

Recommended Affirmations: 2, 16, 21, 26–27 and 30

Reiki Positions: Full-body Reiki with at least five extra minutes at the afflicted area and at A7 (with both hands at the back), B1 (for twenty minutes), B3, B6, C3, C6, D5 and D7 (both variations). Balance the chakras and give extra time to the root and third-eye chakras.

- For cancer involving the mouth or tongue: the soles of the feet.
- For cancer involving the breasts or reproductive or urological tract: full-body treatment with extra time at B6, B7, C2, C5, and D7.
- Chemotherapy burns and splinters the auric field and releases thick, dull, dirty bioplasmic residues that slow the field's functioning. Chemotherapy also adversely affects the functioning of healthy neighbouring cells, releasing harmful waste into the tissues. All these waste products and side effects can be addressed by providing Reiki a few hours before and after treatment. In addition to full-body Reiki, spend extra time at B1 (T variation), B3, B5, B7 and D5, preferably with symbols.

Dietary and Other Suggestions:

For general prevention and healing:

- Adopt a diet rich in fibre and low in fat. Do not let fat exceed one-third of your total caloric intake, as a fatty diet can factor heavily in colon and rectal cancer.

- Eat plenty of dark-green vegetables, cruciferous vegetables such as broccoli, Brussels sprouts, kale, cabbage, cauliflower, watercress, sweet potatoes, tomatoes, ginger, onions, garlic, yoghurt and green peppers.

- Get plenty of beta carotene (carrots, citrus fruits), vitamin A (carrots, apricots mangoes, papayas, spinach), vitamin C (citrus fruits, gooseberries, black currants), vitamin E (whole-grain cereals, cold-pressed vegetable oils such as safflower oil, nuts, eggs, olive oil, avocados, sunflower seeds), vitamin B6 (whole grains, yeast extract, wheat germ, oats, leafy green vegetables, bananas, pulses, dried figs, sunflower seeds), riboflavin (milk, whole-grain cereals, yeast extract), folate (whole-grain cereals, leafy green vegetables, beans, eggs, fruit, peanuts, yeast extract) and selenium (whole-grain cereals, fish, shellfish, fish oils, brewer's yeast).

To *treat most kinds of cancer:*

- Drink a glass of cauliflower juice on an empty stomach every morning.

- Drink a glass of gooseberry juice or eat a sizable quantity of dried gooseberries four times a day.

- Drink a glass of wheat-grass juice thrice a day.

- Drink a glass of carrot juice thrice a day for several months. It is especially beneficial for blood and stomach cancer.

- For stomach cancer, drink some garlic juice in water every day for a few weeks.

- Eat some cooked green turnip tops, or drink their juice, thrice a day.

- Fast for three days. (Have an enema if required.) After three days, start living on grapes alone, up to two kilograms a day. After a week or so, add buttermilk to your diet. You may experience pain in the stomach or anus, but this should not cause concern; it will disappear on its own. Provide Reiki or use a hot pack for relief. The benefits of this regime may take months.

- Mothers should breastfeed their infants to reduce the risk of breast cancer later in life.

- Cut down on animal fats (high beef intake has been linked to cancer of the colon), hydrogenated vegetable oils (including margarine), sugars of all kinds, caffeine, dairy products (except yoghurt), foods with additives, peanuts, smoked or salt-preserved foods (they contain nitrates and nitrites that react with food to form nitrosamines, which cause stomach cancer) and charred, deep-fried, salty, grilled and barbequed foods. Never eat burnt food. Avoid bacon, salt cured and salt-pickled foods (especially pickled fish and cured meats) as these can cause cancer of the mouth, oesophagus and stomach.
- Cut out smoking (in addition to causing lung cancer, it contributes to many other kinds) and alcohol, as they deplete vitamin-B reserves that are essential in fighting cancer. Regular drinking may also increase the risk of cancer of the mouth, throat, oesophagus, stomach, liver, colon and breast.
- Do not sunbathe without protection, as ultraviolet light can cause skin cancer.
- Lose any excess weight. Breast, uterine and gall-bladder cancer are more common among overweight people.
- Imagine that your powerful immune cells are tracking down and killing weak and confused cancer cells. Follow this up with half an hour of deep meditation.
- Have more of the colour gold in your surroundings. Wear gold more often, and meditate on gold for ten minutes daily.

To *prevent specific kinds of cancer*:
- Brussels sprouts, broccoli, cabbage, soybeans and soy products, miso and tofu reduce the risk of breast cancer.
- Fish oil may reduce the risk of breast, bowel, colon and pancreatic cancer.
- Rice, bran, bread and green bananas may reduce the risk of bowel and stomach cancer.
- Kohlrabi (*gaanth gobi*) and turnips are a good source of fibre and thus can help fend off colon and rectal cancer.
- Yoghurt and parsnips may guard against colon cancer.

OTHER PROBLEMS

Accidents

Accidents do not happen to us—they are caused, and often by none other than our own self. Accidents usually take place when you are conflicted, usually unconsciously, about rebelling against authority. Usually this conflict arises in people who find it difficult to speak up for themselves, and who thus let resentment bottle up. Through injury and pain, accidents jolt you into questioning the wisdom of your current course of action. A little analysis, followed by silence, may reveal the underlying conflict. Suppressed anger, guilt, self-pity, frustrations, grave dissatisfaction or rebellion against authority express themselves as accidents that get us the pain, sympathy and attention we are secretly craving.

Recommended Affirmations: 7, 16 and 22–25

Reiki Positions: Call for immediate medical aid if necessary. Then provide Reiki to B2–B3, B5–B6, D5 and the affected areas (keeping your hands away from fresh injuries).

- For those prone to accidents, provide Reiki to the root chakra for twenty extra minutes daily.

Dietary and Other Suggestions: If you are prone to accidents, major or minor, do the following exercises regularly.

Sit down in padmasana. Close your eyes and meditate on the beautiful reds and oranges of the sky at sunset. Imagine these colours permeating your being, and then engulfing your whole body.

Now unlock your legs from padmasana. Extend your right leg straight ahead and bend your left leg at the knee so that your left foot is adjacent to your right knee. Without moving the left foot, drag your right foot back to meet it and let your knees fall down to the sides, as far as they can go. Clasp your hands around your feet. While exhaling, start bending your head forward to meet your feet, stopping when you feel a mild tension. Hold this position for five to ten slow, easy, deep breaths. Slowly resume the original position while breathing in. Repeat five times.

Allergies

An allergy is the body's reaction to a foreign substance it does not like. The most common airborne allergies are house dust, pollen, pet dander and mould. The substance to which you are allergic symbolizes something you are avoiding or suppressing in your life, so you need to identify this facet of your life and integrate it on a conscious level. Spend some time in solitude and quietly notice your resistance, fear or anger.

Recommended Affirmations: 1, 3, 5, 7–8, 16, 22, 25 and 34
Reiki Positions: Full-body treatment followed by extra time at the affected area and at A1–A6 (and the top of the head), B2–B7, C2–C7, D5 (for about half an hour daily) and D7.
Dietary and Other Suggestions:

- Adopt a wholesome vegetarian diet.
- Cover your nose and mouth with a thin cloth while you dust, vacuum or garden. Keep an ionizer switched on indoors, especially while you sleep.
- Avoid wall-to-wall carpeting. Roll up your carpet once a week to clean the floor beneath it, and get the carpet itself washed or dry-cleaned at least twice a year. Washable rugs are preferable.
- Keep your pets out of your bedroom.
- If possible, get yourself an air conditioner and seal the house: it filters the air and keeps the humidity level low. The same holds true for your car.

Childhood Diseases

Childhood diseases, especially those involving the skin, indicate the ushering in of a new phase in the life of the child that calls for resolving a conflict on the part of the child. They also represent the immature and childish behaviour of the people around the child. What the child needs during these times is a lot of attention and love, which can be given, among other ways, in the form of full-body Reiki.

Recommended Affirmation: 13
Reiki Positions: A1–A7 and B1–B6.
Dietary and Other Suggestions: Mix the juices of basil leaves

and garlic in honey and administer a spoonful to the child. Regular use may act as a preventive medicine for children's diseases.

Death (Transition)

Even when Reiki decides that a person cannot be saved from death, it may allow him or her to die peacefully, with minimal pain. Treat the person in transition by channelling Reiki at B1 (heart) and providing mental absentee healing both to him or her and to those who are near and dear.

Fainting

Fainting results from an inadequate supply of oxygen. Standing up too quickly (especially if one is old and weak), standing too long in one position, or anything that suddenly causes the blood pressure to drop (fatigue, pain, emotional upset, shock) may temporarily cut off the supply of oxygen to the brain and result in fainting. Recurrent fainting may indicate a serious underlying problem such as anaemia, diabetes, heart disease or a circulation disorder, and should be thoroughly investigated medically. Metaphysically, fainting manifests a lack of inner strength and some apprehensions about managing something in one's life. Trust in life—let yourself flow lovingly with life as it unfolds before you.

Recommended Affirmations: 2–3, 7–9, 18 and 26–28
Reiki Positions: D7, C2 and C5
Dietary and Other Suggestions:

- Apply pressure with a fingernail on the midlines between the top lip and the nose, two-thirds of the way up.
- When treating others: lay the patient down on his or her back, with legs propped up slightly so as to restore the blood supply to the brain. Ensure that no tight clothing or anything else contricts the air passages in the neck, mouth or chest. If the patient does not revive, turn him or her on his or her side and call for medical assistance.

Fatigue/Weakness

Fatigue is one of the most prevalent health problems. It has many causes: illness, lack of sleep, anaemia, unwholesome diet (especially one low in iron, high in sugar and lacking in essential vitamins and minerals), glandular fever, Myalgic Encephalomyelitis (ME), hormonal imbalance, poor breathing habits, a tendency to worry, a lack of purpose in life, a recent trauma, lack of physical exercise, stress, depression and inability to express emotions (which leads to bottled-up anger, grief, guilt and other negative states). Metaphysically, stress shows an unconscious will to get the rest your body so badly needs.

Recommended Affirmations: 7, 8, 18 and 19

Reiki Positions: Five minutes at A1–A2, A5, A7 (with both hands at the back), B2–B7, C3, C6, D5 and D7 (both variations). Balance the chakras.

Dietary Suggestions: See the sections on breakfast, lunch and dinner in 'Reiki and Diet', Chapter 3.

- For breakfast, have low-fat yoghurt, low-fat milk or paneer, cooked oatmeal or whole-wheat bread, or raisins and cinnamon. Avoid doughnuts, pastries, buttered toast and fried eggs. Avoid heavy meals at midday; soups and fruit or vegetable salads are light and nutritious. Follow lunch with a twenty-minute walk and a forty-minute nap.

- Eat smaller meals more often—four to six times a day. Eat the two major meals before 2 p.m., and insert smaller meals of fresh fruits, raisins, nuts or light high-protein snacks between them.

- Have dinner three hours before you go to bed at night.

- Drink ten to twelve glasses of water each day.

- Drink half a glass of water mixed with a teaspoon of lemon juice and two teaspoons of honey once a day.

- Drink some carrot juice stirred with wheat-grass juice and lemon juice thrice a day.

- Adopt a wholesome vegetarian diet. Whole-meal flour, pulses and oat products provide a slow, steady supply of energy. Eat plenty of low-fat dairy products, yeast extract, wheat germ, fresh and dried fruits, leafy dark-green vegetables and soya products. Take in their natural form, or in supplements, under a physician's guidance, plenty of:

- Vitamin C (citrus fruits, gooseberries, black currants).
- Vitamin B6 (whole grains, yeast extract, wheat germ, oats, green leafy vegetables, bananas, pulses, dried figs sunflower seeds).
- Folic acid (green vegetables, fresh fruits, brewer's yeast or yeast extract, wheat germ, pulses, liver, kidneys, meat).
- Potassium (potatoes, whole-meal flour, cereals, prunes, milk, fresh fruits and vegetables, meat, chicken).
- Zinc (egg yolk, dairy products, whole-grain flour, lentils, nuts, chickpeas, whole-grain cereals and products, shellfish, poultry and lean meat).
- Magnesium (whole-meal flour, whole-grain cereals and products, milk, eggs, meat, nuts, especially Brazil nuts, pulses, dried fruits including figs, garlic, wheat-grass juice, parsley, leafy green vegetables, shellfish, chicken).
- Folate (leafy dark-green vegetables, beans, eggs, fruits, nuts, especially peanuts, yeast extract, whole-grain cereals, liver).
- Vitamin B12 (grapenuts, fortified corn flakes, mushrooms, milk, cheese, dairy products, yeast, meat, liver, kidneys, fish, egg yolk).
- Iron (beans, lentils, nuts, leafy green vegetables, wheat germ, sunflower seeds, meat, liver).
- Complex starchy carbohydrates such as pasta.
- Give up alcohol, smoking, chocolate, tea and coffee. Cut down on sugar, cakes, biscuits and other sweets.
- Gradually lose any excess weight.
- Avoid medicines unless you are sure you need them.

Other Suggestions:

Ensure that you are getting adequate sleep. For ten days, try to go to sleep by nine and do not get up until you awaken naturally. This will reveal your natural sleep requirement. (Ignore the first three days, as they may be influenced by the backlog of sleep-deprivation.) Note that when trying to make up for lost sleep, it is more important to go to bed early than to get up late. An early bedtime is one of the most important habits you can adopt in life: apart from bringing the body more in tune with Nature, it ensures a stress-free early rising. This, in turn, prevents a mad morning rush—the major source of fatigue and absent-mindedness.

- Exercise, do deep-breathing exercises and meditate regularly. Spend fifteen minutes a day on each of the following three: (a) brisk walking, climbing steps, riding an exercise bike, yoga with Surya Namaskar or tai chi; (b) Sudarshan Kriya and proper breathing; (c) yoga nidra or meditation. Try to spread your exercise schedule across the day rather than do everything at one time; in particular, take five-minute breaks for deep breathing several times a day. Avoid strenuous exercise within three to four hours after a meal.
- Have regular massages.
- Apply pressure to the spot where your middle finger rests on your palm when you fold your fingers.
- Soak your legs in a bucket of warm hot water mixed with a tablespoon of salt.
- Install an ionizer in your bedroom and office.
- If possible, take a shower when you feel tired. If not, just splash some cold water on your face.
- Try reading instead of watching television, especially late in the evening.
- Get yourself checked for anaemia and take treatment if necessary.
- Ask yourself whether you find meaning in life. Are you involved in things that are spiritually and emotionally satisfying to you? If not, find a way to start doing something you love every day, whether at work or afterwards.
- Discover your purpose in life by finding out what will give you immense pleasure and what is it that you are likely to be remembered for. Set yearly, monthly, weekly and daily goals towards fulfilling this purpose—each morning, plan the day so that you control (rather than get controlled by) your routine. It is more important to do 'important' things than 'urgent' ones. Powerful goals release energy within you. Think positive, be confident and feel motivated, and

remember that meaningless routine jobs and impotent goals sap this motivation away. Make being happy, healthy and energetic your number one goal in life. In order to accomplish this you have to start respecting your body: listen to it more often, and when it wants to rest, let it rest.

- Close your eyes and think of things that are symbols of energy—strong winds, a running deer or cheetah, a locomotive—and imagine yourself to be a symbol of energy, too. Tell yourself that you are energy personified. Fake it till you make it.
- Go on vacation just to enjoy yourself once a year.
- Resolve any problems in your relationships or the job. Sublimate your negative emotions into a useful activity. Learn to express your feelings, or at least get in touch with them by thinking about them and then letting them dissipate. Try writing them down on a piece of paper and then tearing the paper up.
- Learn to be assertive, and say 'no' to excessive or unnecessary demands on your time and energy.
- Play music that energizes you. You may have to experiment to see what works best.
- Look at the colour red for a little while; it may give you energy. Surround yourself with bright colours in both your home and your workplace, especially reds and greens.

Fever

Fever is a symptom of several diseases, indicating that the body is fighting infection: raising the temperature helps kill invading bacteria. Because of this, it is not advisable to try to lower the body's temperature unless it gets too high—say, beyond 103 degrees F (39 degrees C).

Metaphysically, it is really your anger that is trying to attract your conscious attention. When you have a fever, you should stay in bed and try to identify the underlying reasons for this anger, remembering that sometimes latent excitement has the same effects as unexpressed anger.

Recommended Affirmation: 16

Reiki Positions: Five minutes each at A1 (on the sides of the nose), A3–A6, B1–B3, B5 and D5.

- If the fever is very high or has lasted a long time, follow the above positions with full-body treatment and extra time on C3, C6, D5 and D7 (both variations).

Dietary and Other Suggestions:

- Sponge the whole body beginning with the armpits and groin. Wipe it down one area at a time, leaving the rest of the body covered.
- Avoid solid foods. Drink four to six glasses of fruit or vegetable juice each day, especially beet-root and carrot juice. If you are not also vomiting or experiencing diarrhoea, take light, nourishing meals such as soup, custard and bananas.
- Massage the soles of your feet with freshly cut onions. Hold them in position with the help of a foot wrap, which you can replace every few hours.
- Heat some powdered black pepper and some basil leaves in a glass of water and mix in two teaspoons each of ginger juice and honey. Drink this thrice each day.
- Do not overheat your home.

Infection

An infection is a disease caused by bacteria, a virus or any other micro-organism. Infections draw your attention to a conflict (often attended by irritation, anger or anguish) that you have been refusing to address consciously. The infected organ or body part indicates the kind of the conflict you are running from. Every problem comes into your life to teach you something, and leaves you stronger than before. Get into the habit of consciously recognizing and resolving your conflicts; one way is to sit down with pen and paper and try to define your conflict until you can see it precisely. This should be followed by a silent search in which you focus your attention on the heart chakra or solar-plexus chakra. How does it feel there when you visualize yourself taking action to solve your problem? Is the feeling pleasant and encouraging, or is it discouraging?

Recommended Affirmations: 1, 5, 7, 9, 12, 16, 22 and 24–26

Reiki Positions: To strengthen general resistance to infection, provide Reiki for five minutes at A1 (on the sides of the nose), A7 (with both hands at the back), B3–B4, B7, D7 and at the perineum.

Dietary and Other Suggestions:

- Give up alcohol, chocolate, and coffee.
- Adopt a vegetarian diet, and replace refined sugar and white flour with jaggery and whole-wheat flour.
- Take one garlic clove with every meal.

Influenza ('The Flu')

The flu is a contagious viral infection that cannot be killed by antibodies, as it continually changes and develops new strains. Loss of appetite, fever, chills, shivering, coughing, headache, aching joints, aching muscles, fatigue and general malaise are some of its symptoms. Influenza is a manifestation of excessive stress or a crisis you may be trying to turn your back on. Everyday problem holds the seeds of growth, so you must thank the universe for giving it to you, and then try to resolve it.

Recommended Affirmation 12 and 29

Reiki Treatment: Full-body Reiki with five extra minutes at A7, B1–B2, B7, C3, C6 and the wrists.

Dietary and Other Suggestions:

- Eat small, light meals such as whole-meal bread or cereal. Eat plenty of carrots, apples, garlic, spinach and broccoli. Drink lots of fluids, especially fresh fruit juices and vegetable soups.
- Mix one teaspoon honey, half a teaspoon powdered black pepper, half a teaspoon lemon juice and some basil leaves into a glass of hot water and drink it each morning.
- Take carrot and beet-root juice mixed with an equal quantity of water thrice a day.
- Keep yourself warm. Stay at home until at least a day after the fever subsides, resting completely.
- If you get the flu recurrently, give up smoking.
- If you have headaches or nasal congestion, soak your feet in a bucket of warm water. Use a hot pack on aching muscles.

- Take a steam bath with eucalyptus oil to fight both infection and nasal congestion.
- Do not administer aspirin to children.

Insomnia

Insomnia is as common as the common cold. Lack of sleep makes us irritable, inefficient and unable to concentrate. Most of us undermine our sleep requirements, which can be as high as nine hours, or even more for creative people. Anxiety, stress, pain, late-night heavy meals or coffee, an irregular schedule, depression and obesity can all make it difficult to sleep. Try going to bed fifteen minutes earlier every week until you are retiring an hour earlier by the end of the month, and see if this raises your alertness level during the day. If so, add more intervals of fifteen minutes until you are sure you have found your real sleep requirement. No physical exercise, breathing technique or meditation can help you if your body is starved of sleep. Many people wonder for years what is wrong with them— they feel tired and absent-minded every day—and they try clinical tests, new diets and exercise without ever realizing that the problem is simple sleep deprivation.

Metaphorically speaking, falling asleep is a voluntary act of letting yourself go and welcoming the unknown future (akin to what is required to die peacefully and gracefully). Those who feel guilty about their past or worry too much about their future find it difficult to undertake these everyday rehearsals for their ultimate death. Learn to express your feelings in a constructive manner, and find solutions to your problems rather than simply worrying about them.

Recommended Affirmations: 2, 4, 7 and 30
Reiki Positions:

- Five minutes each at A1–A2, B1–B2, B4, B6–B7, C3 and C7.
- Place one hand at B2 and the other at A5, support your arms on pillows and fall asleep this way.

Dietary Suggestions:

- Do not smoke, eat chocolate or drink alcohol, cola or coffee after 4 p.m. They will interfere with your ability to fall asleep.

- Avoid late-night meals, especially spicy, heavy, greasy or rich ones. However, do not go to bed hungry, either; eat pasta, rice or potatoes in the evening.

- If you suffer from restless legs—involuntary movements of the leg muscles that can make it difficult to fall asleep—you should treat that condition first. Adopt a diet of iron-rich foods such as pulses, dried apricots, leafy dark-green vegetables and nuts, especially almonds.

- Eat dinner early, preferably by 7 p.m. (at least three hours before your bedtime), and go for an evening stroll.

- Before going to bed, take any of the following: some fresh lettuce or an apple, a glass of onion juice, yoghurt mixed with black pepper, sugar and aniseed, some coriander paste with a little sugar, toast with jam or a glass of milk. The latter may not suit some people because of its protein content; add a little saffron and see if it works for you.

***Other Suggestions*:**

- Soak your calves in a bucket of warm water for five minutes before going to bed. (In summer you can use room-temperature water.)

- Massage your feet with mustard oil at bedtime.

- Do not put off going to bed. Follow a strict regimen of going to bed and getting up at fixed hours, including weekends.

- Follow a daily regimen of physical exercise, breathing exercise and meditation. Include some non-strenuous exercise such as walking. If you work in an office, take a warm shower as soon as you get home. Do not exercise late in the evening.

- If you take an afternoon nap, limit it to one hour and be done with it by 3 p.m.

- Evening is a time to wind down, but some of us refuse to do so, carrying on with our work, TV viewing or computer activities till late at night. This is the time to do light things such as listening to soothing music, light reading or spending time with your family or friends.

- Keep your bedroom at the right temperature, neither too cold nor too hot, and keep it dark and well ventilated.

- Try sex when you find it hard to fall asleep.
- If you work in shifts try to stick to the same one, or arrange for the shifts to change in a forward direction. That is, change from a morning shift to a midday shift to a night shift rather than mixing things up.
- Stop worrying about your insomnia; that will only worsen it.
- Do not take crossword puzzles, office work, worries or anything that taxes your mind to bed. Go to bed only when you really mean to sleep.
- If you wake up in the middle of the night, do not get up and start working or moving around. Just stay in bed and pay close attention to your breathing, or imagine that you are climbing down a staircase one step at a time (while counting) or start giving yourself Reiki. Some low, soothing music may help, including music recorded with natural sounds such as those of flowing water or bird calls. Shift your focus from stressful thoughts to beautiful memories.
- Save an hour before you go to sleep for reviewing the day's activities backwards, from evening to morning. Do not justify or condemn any of your actions; conclude by focusing on your concerns, guilt, worries and any other problems at hand, and the lessons learnt from the day.

Malaria

Malaria is caused by the bite of a female mosquito, which injects its saliva before sucking some blood. (The mosquito itself gets infected by sucking the blood of a person carrying parasites.) Symptoms may take from twelve days to ten months to appear. Metaphysically, malaria reminds us of the need to regain balance in our lives.

Recommended Affirmations: 7, 16 and 22–25
Reiki Positions: Full-body treatment with extra time on B2–B4 and B6.
Dietary and Other Suggestions:

- To prevent malaria, chew some betel leaves every morning on an empty stomach.

- To treat malaria: mix twenty basil leaves and ten black peppers into some sugary boiled water and drink a glass every day.

- Grind sixty grams of neem leaves and four black peppers, boil them in a cup of water and drink the mixture once a day.

- Suck a lemon sprinkled with powdered black pepper powder and salt. Mix two teaspoons of lemon juice and some honey into a glass of water and drink the mixture every morning for a week.

- Boil the peels of two oranges in two cups of water until the water is down to one cup. Strain and drink once a day.

- Before the onset of fever, mix one teaspoon each of garlic juice and sesame oil, and suck this paste every hour for four days.

- Before the onset of fever, grind a teaspoon of unroasted caraway seeds, mix them with a little jaggery and roll them into three tiny globules. Eat these hourly for four days.

- Eat plenty of apples and guavas, especially before the onset of fever.

- Once you have a fever, drink a glass of buttermilk every fourth day.

Motion Sickness

Motion sickness is the nausea and/or headache that some people suffer when travelling. It is caused by a conflict between what the eyes see and what the inner ear feels during the journey: though the eyes adapt to the movement, the ears do not, and the mixed signals sent to the brain result in nausea.

Metaphysically, motion sickness represents a feeling of being trapped, and unease with having to let go of the familiar and accept a new future. Be curious about what lies ahead, and trust that it can only be in your ultimate favour because the universe holds nothing less than that for you. Seasickness represents fear of death or a feeling of lack of control.

Recommended Affirmations: 2, 4 and 6–9
Reiki Positions: A2–A3, A5–A6 and B3

Dietary and Other Suggestions:

- Get plenty of sleep before the trip.
- Before and during the journey, chew a few pieces of peeled fresh ginger. At the first signs of nausea, suck a lemon sprinkled with salt.
- Take plenty of water and fluids such as fresh fruit juices (take the fruit itself if you are not sure about the quality of the juice) before and during the journey.
- Do not eat large meals or drink alcohol before or during the journey.
- If you are prone to motion sickness, try to travel at night.
- Do not smoke during the trip, and avoid passive smoke as well. Keep your head still, and postpone reading. If you must read, hold the page close to eye level and turn your back on the window.
- Fix your sight on a stationary object in the distance, on land or in the sky. When travelling in a car, sit in the front and watch the road ahead or the horizon. If possible, stop the car and take fresh-air breaks every so often, complete with deep-breathing exercises.
- Press the point in the centre of the forearm that is in line with the middle finger, three fingers' width from the wrist-palm joint crease.

Nails

Nail-biting often results from anxiety, tension or insecurity and may weaken the nails or damage the sensitive skin underneath. Nails represent protection, so nail-biting shows a lack of confidence, a need to defend oneself and parental pressure to conform to expectations. By biting the nails, a child is unconsciously trying to bolster his or her self-confidence.

Recommended Affirmations: 7, 16 and 22–29

Reiki Positions: Full-body Reiki with extra time on D7.

Dietary and Other Suggestions:

- Paint the nails with a bitter-tasting polish, sold by chemists for this purpose.
- Improve self-esteem and security through counselling.

- Eat plenty of foods rich in iron, zinc and vitamin C. Avoid tea.
- White spots on the nails are due to a deficiency of zinc and vitamin A (not calcium), and can be rectified with spinach, sunflower seeds and zinc-rich foods or zinc supplements. Zinc also prevents brittle nails, infections of the surrounding skin, and thin, spoon-shaped nails, especially on the thumbs
- To relieve whitlows (abscesses), wear rubber gloves when working with water.
- Apply hand cream regularly, especially after drying the hands, to avoid brittle or splitting nails.
- Soften the nails in warm water before trimming them. Cut them in a straight line only.

Pain

Pain is the body's way of drawing your attention to something that needs to be healed. It often prevents further injury, as when you are burned by a sharp stove or pricked by a sharp object. Sometimes pain is felt not at the site of the problem but elsewhere; this is known as referred pain. (For example, heart disorders are often felt in the left arm and fingers.)

The type of pain represents the type of malady. Continuous throbbing pain indicates an inflammation. Continuous dull pain indicates strained muscles or ligaments. Intermittent stabbing pain indicates the stretching or swelling of a tube-like part of the body, such as the intestine. Burning pain indicates tissue damage due to heat, friction or chemicals.

Metaphysically, pain follows a hindrance to the flow of life because of accumulated repressed feelings, usually some kind of guilt. The area or part of the body that is giving you pain reflects the psychological part of your being that is yearning to be freed or integrated with the rest. If you feel your pain with full attention, rather than trying to run from it, the pain will soon be on its way out, as its very purpose was to draw your attention. Learn to let go of those aspects of your emotional self that need to be liberated (for example, a need for self-punishment stemming from guilt).

Recommended Affirmations: 2, 7 and 30
Reiki Positions: The top of the shoulders (the soft spot next to the bone).
Dietary and Other Suggestions:

- Drink lots of fluids.
- Eat plenty of pumpkin and sesame seeds, bananas, avocados, lima beans, peanuts, almonds, cheese and herring. The body uses these to produce pain-killing hormones.
- If you do not have diabetes or heart disease, apply an ice pack to the pain, taking intermittent breaks. You may also try a hot pack, but do not switch abruptly between the two.
- If you have an injured limb, prop it up to keep it above the level of the heart.
- Relax with yoga nidra.
- Imagine that a misty cloud of healing energy is gathering around the painful area and permeating it. Imagine that it is repairing the injured cells and bringing great relief. Imagine your individual cells smiling with the ensuing happiness.

Shock

Clinical shock results from insufficient blood supply to vital organs such as the brain and kidneys. It occurs after burns, accidents, extreme pain or distress, vomiting, diarrhoea, blood infection or severe allergies and requires immediate medical attention. Symptoms may include grey, cold and moist skin, fast, shallow breathing, a weak, fast pulse, dizziness, faintness, blurred vision, thirst, anxiety, restlessness and sometimes unconsciousness.

Recommended Affirmations: 7, 16 and 22–25
Reiki Positions: Until medical help arrives, provide Reiki at the wrists, B6, B1, the ends of the shoulders and D5. Later on, provide full-body treatment with extra time at A1–A2, A4–A5, B2, B6–B7, C3, C6, D5 and D7.
Dietary and Other Suggestions:

- Lay the patient down, prop up his or her legs and keep the head below the level of the heart. If the patient is unconscious, have him or her lie on the stomach with the face to one side.

- Loosen the clothing around the neck, chest and waist.
- If the patient complains of thirst, do not give him or her anything to drink; just moisten his lips with water.
- Assure the patient that he or she is safe and you are not leaving him or her unattended.

Side Effects of Antibiotics
Recommended Affirmations: 7
Reiki Positions: Full-body treatment every other day for two weeks, then daily for another few days on A6, B1, B3, B6, C2–C7 and D5.
Dietary and Other Suggestions: Antibiotics destroy beneficial bacteria in the gut. Eating live yogurt helps restore them.

Stammering
Stammering is a very common speech problem. It may stem from over-anxious parents, an emotional shock or distressing experience suffered in early childhood or slow development of the coordination of tongue, palate and lips. Metaphysically, stammering reveals your efforts to hide feelings of insecurity. Spend some time in silence every day, get in touch with your thoughts and feelings and accept them totally, with deep love, without condemning or justifying them. Accept yourself as you are.
Recommended Affirmations: 10
Reiki Positions: A6 and B4
Dietary and Other Suggestions:

- Sit erect in a chair, and raise your arms while inhaling and then holding your breath. Breathe out slowly while bringing your arms down. Now speak fluently.
- Press down on the bottom outside corner of your thumbnail for a minute. Release and repeat five times. Do this many times each day.
- Practise singing.
- Try hypnotherapy.

5

The Spirit of Reiki: Living the Five Principles

Becoming a Reiki channel is the beginning of your journey back to yourself, not the end of it. Reiki may bring hidden facets of your personality to the fore so that you can address them responsibly, but it also leaves you with the freedom to ignore them or act irresponsibly. That is why Reiki is only one tool for personal transformation. It needs to be accompanied by your commitment to five definite principles that will fine-tune your life with cosmic intelligence. Dr Mikao Usui, the re-discoverer of Reiki, adopted these principles to support healing sessions and make them more effective.

The beauty of these principles is that they flow into each other, and facilitate their collective integration into one's life. Each principle begins with the words 'Just for today', emphasizing that we need to live life one day at a time with complete attention. Dr Usui was aware that committing to something for the rest of one's life is intimidating, sometimes to the point of discouraging one even from attempting it. Anyone who takes these principles seriously and consciously makes them a part of his or her personality is bound to be blessed by the very Reiki energy itself.

THE FIRST PRINCIPLE OF REIKI

Just for today, I shall live the attitude of gratitude.

Gratitude is the heart's acknowledgement of the song of love that the universe is, and to our beautiful and sacred relationship to it. It is the heart's appreciation of Nature's generosity, and of God's immense love for us, which he has shown by making us from the same stuff He himself is made up of—the same seamless One spirit—and hence accepting us unconditionally and eternally as part of Him.

Consciously or unconsciously, we often pray and ask God or the universe to materialize our desires. God listens even to the wishes of atheists, who prefer to send their prayers without naming the receiver, knowing deep within that all wishes are directed only to Him and need not be addressed formally to Him. However, when wishes are granted and we retrace with loving gratitude the channels through which we sent our prayers, we feel complete, and connected to the completeness of the universe.

Why should we live the attitude of gratitude?

With gratitude, happiness comes on its own. One reason we lead very ordinary lives in spite of being children of God is the fact that we seek what we are already surrounded with. If we only look within and around ourselves more consciously, we realize that we are swimming in a sea of blessings. *When we focus our attention not on what we have but on what we do not have, our happiness is eternally postponed to the future.* When, instead, we focus on what we have, we get ideas on how to use it more creatively to get what we still want. *Instead of focusing on what is missing from your life—money, a car, a house, a good relationship*—feel deep gratitude for all the comforts and good things the Latent Oneness has already blessed you with. If you do so, these things will multiply, and you will not make yourself miserable by dwelling on what you don't have.

Make a list of all that you have achieved in your life. Every time you achieve a goal, add it to your list of achievements. Think of the things that were once your most cherished desires— things you hoped to do, to learn, to become, to purchase, people you hoped to befriend or love—and note how many *are* realities today. Think also of the body parts that have been serving you since your birth: remember that not every body is blessed with hands or feet. You are one of the fortunate ones. Read this list every day and thank God for everything on it. Working for and getting what you seek without taking time to feel grateful for it is like sowing the seeds and nurturing the plants but never bothering to reap the harvest. With gratitude, the cycle of happiness is complete.

There will always be things we do not have or have not yet become. The world is full of people who find reasons to postpone being happy. They are just not in the habit of being happy, and some are not even sure it's okay to feel happy. Some of us, because of childhood conditioning, feel guilty aiming for happiness; others are afraid it might bring sorrow in its wake.

Most of us do not realize that getting what we aspire to will not necessarily make us happy. Achieving, becoming or possessing something does not necessarily mean feeling happy about it. Thus, for most of us happiness remains an eternal chase—a mirage.

Happiness is also the difference between sleepwalking through life and being consciously aware of the joys of life, from moment to moment. Truly happy people are happy within their everyday contexts; they do not seek the 'rush' of big moments. Life is too short to wait for big moments.

If you want abundance to flow in your life, let gratitude flow in your blood. Whatever we give our thoughts to, expands—so you should always focus on abundance, never on scarcity. No economic strategies can ever remove poverty from the face of this planet because poverty does not come from without. Can you change an image in the mirror without changing the object itself? And if not, how can you change poverty without changing the attitudes and belief systems of the poor? The first step towards transforming poverty into riches is to encourage the poor person to shift his attention from what he lacks to what he possesses—even if that is only an aluminum utensil. The next step is to make him realize how he would feel without these possessions, and hence that he should feel grateful to the universe for arranging it for him. The third step is to think of those who do not possess even these things, and pray that they, too, be blessed with this and much more. The fourth step is to believe in abundance and live life according to this belief. In other words, start thinking, living and behaving like a rich man.

If this principle often fails to manifest the abundance in the world of form, it is only because of our limiting beliefs—just as the kitchen bulb fails to give full illumination because of the smoke accumulated on it, even when the filament is producing good light. Instead of pitying the poor, pray sincerely that through God's grace they may come to realize their inner riches so they can see their external riches, too. Abundance is attracted to gratitude.

Affirmations to Develop the Attitude of Gratitude

I thank you (the Latent Oneness underlying the Universe) for letting me work in an area you had planned for me. I thank you for all the material things, skills and talents you have given me, and also for the love you have given me through various manifestations on the material plane.

- I thank you for giving me a house to live in, a cause to work for, a means by which to commute to work, a family with whom to share my love, money for my material needs, and the peace to experience Your bliss.
- I thank You for fulfilling my personal goals of the past, present and future.
- I thank You for the sad occasions I have experienced, as they taught me lessons I needed to learn.

What keeps us from living the attitude of gratitude?

We take things for granted, and find reasons to be sad rather than reasons to be happy. Taking things for granted desensitizes you to the beauty of life. If you think of the joys, learning experiences and comforts you would lose without the people and things presently in your life, you will realize the ocean of blessings and gifts in which you live, and your heart will swell with gratitude.

Our focus is more on complaining, blaming and finding fault with others than on what others have done for us. Instead of taking responsibility for ourselves, seeing our own shortcomings and learning from them we tend to believe that all our discomforts and misfortunes are the fault of others. Such an attitude naturally makes it difficult to be grateful for what others have actually done for us.

How can you cultivate the attitude of gratitude?

Instead of finding reason to complain or blame, find love. Whenever you feel like criticizing someone or something, shift your focus to finding what is good in it. If you find this difficult, think of the process as an act of God's love. When you challenge, criticize or blame anyone or anything, you are, in fact, trying to confront God. A complaining nature indicates that you are still in the vice-like grip of your ego—which is, by its very nature, insatiable. You might feel that the perfect situation is elsewhere, but by assuming so you are disconnecting yourself from your own possibilities for joy, happiness and prosperity. The world is however you find it.

Your complaints do not reflect on the things you are complaining about; they reflect on you, indicating that you still lack love in your heart. You are not connected to God, as you still do not trust Him completely.

Catch yourself when you are about to complain or criticize somebody. Instead of finding fault or questioning someone's behaviour, find something that explains it. Imagine yourself to be that person. If you are about to criticise a discourteous waiter, try to get inside the mind of that waiter—ask yourself what might make you behave this way, and remember that you would hope for empathy and understanding in such a situation.

Focus your attention on chance favourable events. The more you do this, the more you become aware of the happy small events that greet you every day. Whenever you receive a compliment, good wishes, an expression of love, a gift or money in any form, give thanks both to the one *through* whom they come and to the One *from* whom they come.

Behind every little thing that makes our lives comfortable or enjoyable are the hidden services of countless people. For instance, I am writing these lines on a personal computer. Countless engineers worked for years with countless associates in many capacities to develop the various software packages and improve the hardware to its present state. Manufacturers, assemblers and transporters made it possible for the computer to reach me. The ideas I am writing down are the results of thoughts I have been able to think, and these thoughts are the result of profound and painstaking contemplation augmented by the inspiration of thousands of known and unknown sages, scientists, authors, great minds and ordinary people. I may have heard about these people through my family, teachers, friends or colleagues, or I may have read about them in books. These books, in turn, are the results of hard work by publishers, editors, artists, printers, binders, distributors, transporters (including drivers who might be illiterate themselves) and booksellers, quite apart from the authors. Each of them must have used gadgets and instruments that, again, were made possible by the contributions of countless other people.

Trust that you are complete and perfect. You lack nothing. If a baby tree compares itself with one that is fully grown, it will naturally feel incomplete, not realizing that it will grow to the same height according to the genetic information in its seed. It can only keep itself from reaching its fullest form by doubting and worrying about it.

Cultivate an attitude of giving. Gratitude and giving grow on each other. A heart bathed in gratitude yearns to give back and serve others. Life passes away very quickly when we are focused on getting, achieving and hoarding, but when we focus on giving, we are filled with meaning and purpose, and the satisfaction of knowing that we are not wasting life.

Paradoxically, when we spend our lives merely receiving and hoarding things or labels, we lose it. A dying man will never tell you that he regrets not having earned more money or a few more promotions. He will probably tell you, with pain in his heart and tears in his eyes, that he did not love or give to others enough.

Use adverse circumstances as the perfect 'laboratory' for attitudes of gratitude and giving. Feeling gratitude is often difficult when things are not going well for us, or in any case not matching our expectations. These are the times when we must trust God and remember that everything He does is done in our best interest.

Prayers are *always* answered. However, we tend to recognize them only when they are answered in the way we requested (and even then, we sometimes dismiss the outcome as sheer coincidence). Gratitude must be felt and offered even when God does not seem to be responding to our prayers, as these are the times when God is protecting us from the wishes and desires that, if fulfilled, would prove disastrous for us. Observe an inner silence and pray for the wisdom to understand the lessons being conveyed in what we are labelling 'unfavourable experience' during these times.

Each brush with adversity leaves you stronger than you were before.

Practice giving during difficult times, too. These are ideal opportunities to be magnanimous, kind, loving, affectionate, caring and understanding with others. If you learn to drive on difficult roads, you become an excellent driver.

THE SECOND PRINCIPLE OF REIKI

Just for today, I shall not worry.

Worrying is a natural reaction to a perceived threat, and has been essential for our survival ever since we appeared on this planet. The positive purpose of worrying is to prepare responses to situations in case they actually arise. Ironically, though, most of the eventualities we worry about have almost no chance of happening, and usually do not take place at all. Even when we worry about things that may happen, we forget the positive purpose of worrying: we dwell on images of the threat rather than solutions to it. When the source of our anxiety is real, the anxiety vanishes when the source is removed; but when the source is a creation of our imagination, the anxiety goes on and on.

Lurking beneath persistent thoughts of impending danger are subconscious warnings that we probably need to look within and confront our guilt, instead of behaving contrary to our values, conscience or the laws of Nature. The hardest misfortunes to bear are those that we create and 'live in' mentally by worrying about them, even though they never actually befall us.

Why do people worry?

Worriers derive false psychological satisfaction from the illusion that worrying about something they dread will keep it from actually happening. Worrying can also hijack one's attention from the present source of worry to another source, ironically bringing 'relief' from the original dreaded prospect by replacing it with another. Compared to visual images, thoughts are poor sources of worry.

Worrying can distract one's attention from the hard work one is not prepared to do to change one's attitude, overcome one's weaknesses and bad habits and bring about change in one's life. It has the added advantage of catching others' attention and drawing their sympathy.

We are conditioned to value our reputation more than our character. Most of our worries pertain to our being accepted by others. Many of us are more interested in others' opinions than in discovering our own values and weaknesses and working on them in order to become what we really want to be.

We do not pay complete attention to our work. If we attend fully to the tasks at hand, the habitual pattern of responses that leads to worry cannot find a free path to flow on.

Many of us breathe very fast. We take quick and shallow breaths that suppress the level of carbon dioxide in the blood. A low level of carbon dioxide constricts the arteries, reducing the flow of blood throughout the body and causing a shortage of oxygen throughout the body. This switches on our sympathetic nervous system, trigger to a worrying disposition.

Why should we stop worrying?

Worrying consumes you physically. Recent research proves beyond a doubt that worry and stress can cause or aggravate angina, arthritis, diabetes, bulimia, cold sores, dandruff, forgetfulness, heartburn, herpes, insomnia, psoriasis, baldness, restless-leg syndrome, ulcers, warts, wrinkles, body odour, hyperventilation and hypertension. Sadly, the worries that cause these diseases are unnecessary, avoidable and serve no positive purpose. Worry does not exist in the external world—we create it by responding to external situations in a self-defeating way. These responses are within our control; we learnt them unconsciously, and we can unlearn them the same way.

Worrying does not help. Everything you worry about turns out the way it was going to, despite your worries—and every moment you spend worrying about it is wasted. Once you know how exquisitely the universe is orchestrated, what can you worry about? Every time we worry instead of preparing calmly for tomorrow, we show that we have yet to believe, trust and surrender to the will of God. We must realize that for the needs of today we have been given corresponding strength but for the needs of tomorrow we can only trust, as tomorrow is not ours yet. Most of our responses in the form of thoughts, speech and action on any given day are the same as yesterday's—

conditioned, repetitive and habit-forming. If you observe them, you will find a definite pattern in the kinds of things you normally worry about.

Worrying often makes dreaded episodes or accidents *more* likely. When you spend your energy imagining negative things, they become more likely to happen. Gurudev Rabindranath Tagore used to say, 'You cannot cross the sea just by staring at the water.' Think about what is needed and do it, instead of just worrying about it. If you can do something to avert, lighten or deal with what you are worrying about, fine. If not, why borrow misery from the future for your bright and beautiful present?

How can you liberate yourself from the habit of worrying?

Believe that being free of all worries is possible. Understand that money, status, intelligence and contacts cannot make you happy. Many people with all of these things live lives of pitiable misery. Being happy takes a lot less energy than making yourself miserable, but you have to learn consciously how to be happy whereas being miserable is an unconscious process. Happiness does not come from external conditions; it comes from your attitude.

Become aware of your pattern of worry. Every time you worry, consider the underlying reason and note it in a diary. Also note the negative adjectives and adverbs you use and underline them. Soon you will see a pattern in what kinds of thoughts trigger anxiety, and this will help you nip them in the bud when they arise and replace them with neutral or positive ones.

Worry at a fixed time every day. This will keep you from worrying during the rest of the day, and will also impress upon you the absurdity of worrying at all. If you have a tendency to get carried away, set an alarm clock to 'wake' you from your worries after ten minutes. During this time, observe and write down all the worries you are currently occupied with or *could* worry about. Sign and date the paper and place it in a folder.

Once a week, review all that you worried about the previous week and write your comments—what have you learned from this review? Eventually, tear the accumulated worry-lists into pieces and throw them into the dustbin.

Get regular exercise and practise relaxation. Physical activity produces chemicals that relax you and make you happy. Get at least half an hour of exercise and half an hour of meditation or relaxation every day. What is most important is regularity, not how much time you devote at a stretch. Yoga, yoga nidra, shavasana, tai chi, massage, meditation and soothing music are all great ways to relax your body. To meditate, sit straight and erect and pay attention to your breath as you exhale and inhale without attempting to change it in any way.

If you have taste for dancing, that could also be a great worry-buster. (Singing also helps!) Another option is to go for a walk, and after every few steps look up towards the sky and feel that you are one with the vast sky and nature.

Take an extra-long bath with soothing music and incense sticks burning near your bathtub. Alternately, soak your feet in warm water and then massage them with sesame or rose oil.

Make yourself laugh several times during the day. Laughter is another great medicine. Laugh, laugh and laugh, even without a reason—the body cannot distinguish between natural and artificial laughter. If you find this difficult, read a joke book, watch a funny film or just put yourself in the company of cheerful people with a good sense of humour.

Challenge your assumptions. 'What makes me think the dreaded event will take place? How valid are my assumptions? What can I do to prevent it from happening? How can I deal with it constructively if it does happen? What is the *worst* that can happen? Is playing and replaying this worry-tape over and over again helping me in any way? If not, why am I doing it?' Ask yourself these questions every time you find yourself being sucked into the anxiety spiral; this will weaken the neural circuitry that supports the worrying pattern.

Imagine that you are a cinema screen. You accept all that is projected on to you without any reaction, knowing well that you remain what you are regardless of what you 'receive'. Accept fear as a part of life, especially the fear that accompanies change. Go ahead, in spite of the pounding heart that seems to call you back. Human beings, unlike comfortable but lazy crocodiles, are meant to live with risk and adventure.

Shift your focus from worrying to finding solutions. Make yourself so busy setting targets and achieving them that you hardly have any time to worry. Ask yourself every morning, 'What is it that I am happy about in my life?' Repeat the question three more times replacing the word 'happy' with 'excited', 'proud' and 'grateful'. In the evening, ask yourself the same questions and consider one worthwhile thing you achieved, contributed or learned today that you can use as an investment in your future. If you know what you want and feel willing and eager to bring it about, you are more likely to get it. We make ourselves weaker by brooding over our weaknesses, and stronger by focusing on our strengths.

Keep your diet natural. Minimize your intake of prepared foods with chemical additives and quick-fix-drugs, especially pain-killers (Do not send the spider in to kill the fly). Drugs do not make you better; they only take away the symptoms for a while. Just as you have unwittingly created the chemicals that have caused you dis-ease by thinking negative thoughts, you can create the chemicals to cure these dis-eases by thinking positive thoughts. And the chemicals you generate from within are free, more effective and have no unpleasant side effects.

Get organized. Do not waste time. Plan your day and stick to it. Set and keep regular hours for everything: work, exercise, breathing, meditation, self-growth, meals and leisure. Do important things first; they do not pressure you the way 'urgent' things do, and attending to important things keeps them from becoming urgent. Think hard before committing yourself and others; every time you break your word you break yourself (your self-esteem) to some extent. If you must break an appointment, inform the other person as soon as possible and discuss the next-best plan of action.

Keep your workstation uncluttered—be ready with

everything you might need for the day's work. If possible, keep a green plant nearby and water it yourself. Keep an ionizer on (do this in your bedroom as well). Wear light-coloured clothes.

Strengthen your second and third chakras. Worrying is exacerbated by dysfunctional second and third chakras (especially the third), which can be strengthened through Reiki. You can also practise the camel posture or ushtrasana, the backward bend—kneel on the floor and move your arms backwards in an arc (one at a time) until your hands rest on the soles of the feet. Your torso should arch outwards like a bow. The spinal twist (ardha matsyendra asana) also strengthens these chakras.

Try these exercises:
- Press the pads of your fingertips gently but firmly together and hold for ten breaths.
- Create a guttural 'Whooooo' sound in the back of the throat.

Train yourself to breathe more slowly. Reach a stage where you are breathing twelve to sixteen times a minute or even less. Remember to involve your abdomen in breathing; abdominal breathing can help alleviate the tendency to worry.

Watch your language. Identify negative verbs such as 'I hate…', 'getting on my nerves', 'I have to', 'I must', 'I should', 'I don't have time' and so forth. Replace them with 'I may', 'I accept', 'I choose to', 'I will find time to' and so forth.

Build relationships. Smile more often, and learn to be polite. Try helping others, including strangers. Be genuinely magnanimous and friendly. Whenever you see anyone, imagine love pouring out of your heart and enveloping him or her. Instead of worrying about your deteriorating relationships and blaming them on others, try to find out what behaviour of yours might have contributed to this deterioration. Instead of wondering whether the other person will ever come to his or her senses and realise his or her mistake, correct what you can in your own behaviour, including the doubt and mistrust through which you now perceive this relationship .

Cut down on reading the crime page, reading crime thrillers

and excessive viewing of TV and movies. You may be letting in too much sorrow and violence in the guise of information and entertainment. We can apply ourselves to problems in our personal lives, but we can do nothing to resolve the tension and anxiety of the characters in movies and soap operas. We accumulate this tension passively.

Notice how you talk to yourself. Do you talk encouragingly or discouragingly? Do you compliment yourself or condemn and abuse yourself? Whenever you talk to yourself, choose positive, empowering, encouraging thoughts.

Tape your dream life in your own voice in vivid detail and listen to it every day (ideally before falling asleep), adding visual and tactile details in your mind's eye. For instance, if you worry about your health, imagine yourself to be extremely healthy; if you worry about money, imagine yourself to be immensely rich.

When reviewing your daily life, step out of the scenes that worry you. Be a spectator to those scenes rather than a participant. Imagine that you are the editor of the movie—turn down the sounds, turn off the colours and make the pictures fainter and smaller until they are lost. With pictures that make you happy, do just the opposite—make them large, colourful, vivid, and well focussed, with clearly audible sounds. Choose your favourite place at home (a chair, a couch or whatever), and before you go and sit there, think of a happy time and enhance its effects as explained above. Go and sit in your favourite place, continue to think of happy times, and when you get up, leave the happy vibrations behind. Do this every day and you will soon find that sitting there makes you feel happy and secure, even blissful. When you are away from home, imagine yourself going to this place and the results will be the same.

Pay attention to the enemy within. You can be your best friend or your worst enemy. Look for things you do every day that make you unhappy or tired. Ask yourself why you do them. Can you find healthier activities that do not have these side effects?

THE THIRD PRINCIPLE OF REIKI

Just for today, I shall not get angry.

Anger often goads us into action. If poor grades, unkind remarks or the sight of injustice make us angry enough to work against them, anger is desirable; just as worry is desirable when it helps us avert a dreaded event. However, anger is often a response to a blocked choice, and projects our displeasure with ourselves. It also reflects our apathy towards the rights of those around us to be free of our hostile attitude.

Why do people get angry?

We are unable to do what we want. Frustration and angry thoughts are our responses to external events that have not taken place according to our expectations. If you planned to read a book this evening but your spouse and children are demanding your attention, you may ultimately lose your temper. Take away expectations and their shadow—anger—disappears, too. Anger has nothing to do with the outside world.

Anger gives a false sense of self-worth. Angry people may feel pleased that, if nothing else, they can produce more anger than others can; they often mistake anger for bravery. People may also show anger to elicit pity for themselves, make others feel guilty or get others to do their bidding.

We feel remorse. Not meeting our own expectations, or feeling bad about our failure to act as we could have to achieve better results, can make us redirect our anger towards others. Someone who performs badly in an important meeting may then scold his or her subordinate for being incompetent. We often redirect anger that we feel towards ourselves or other individuals towards a safer target, rather than confront our low self-esteem and do something about it.

We feel inferior because we are in a vulnerable situation. A contractor reveals your inadequacy in framing the contract agreement; you are losing money and time on a project. You are in a weak legal position, and cannot 'win' this external situation. The only way to show that you are a 'winner' is to display your anger overtly and hurl empty threats at him. People often try to compensate for inner weakness or low self-esteem by projecting power, supremacy or individuality through anger— an immature response.

Anger is also a defensive manoeuver that keeps others from getting too close, both professionally or personally. It seems the easiest way to say, 'Go away'.

To show that you desperately need help. You are packing for an official tour. There is a little time left. You are struggling to fasten the belt on your luggage. After a few unsuccessful attempts, you might lose your patience and shout to someone nearby: 'Don't you see that I am in a hurry and that I need help? Will you please drop everything and help me out?!'

Why should we avoid anger?

We often unleash anger on those who love us most, because anger is the weapon of the weak and cowardly. The weak and cowardly often direct their anger towards soft, safe targets, knowing that the person they are really angry with may be too powerful to confront. Anger is a double-edged sword that damages the targeted person, all beholders and ultimately all of humanity. (Conversely, when you are aware of the underlying reasons for another person's anger, you can respond to the person instead of his undesirable behaviour.)

Anger and hatred can never be overcome by *more* anger and hatred. Hate can *only* be overcome by love and understanding. All that you fight against weakens you, and all that you support strengthens you.

Every moment spent judging or evaluating another person is a moment that deprived you of an opportunity to love someone. You cannot give out anger or hate if you have patience, compassion, understanding and love within. The very reason you exist is to give yourself and your love to others unconditionally, and to receive everything that comes your way with deep gratitude (even if it does not match your expectations).

Every moment you spend being upset over others' behaviour is a moment you choose to be controlled by others.

Nothing consumes a person faster than the flames of a wish to take revenge.

Though anger is as natural to us as colours are to the sky, holding on to it serves no purpose. Some believe that anger is therapeutic, but it is not. Its roots are within us, in the way we process external events, and we alone are responsible for it.

All of your angry thoughts create toxic chemicals that are stored in your body and cause fatigue, pain, stress, anxiety and disease. Whenever you choose between affection and anger, you in fact choose between bodily health and disease. Wherever you see unfavourable circumstances, do not try to change them; changing the mirror will show only what you have made yourself from within. You may see your hair in the mirror, but you comb it where it actually is—on your head.

You have no choice but to accept the various people in your life as they are. Think of a world in which the people have only one face and one personality, the flowers are all of one colour and the trees are all of one kind. The world would be so monotonous, so boring! Thank people different from you for being different. Do not judge—people shall continue to be the way they are in spite of your judgements, anger and hostility. Judging and objecting will only make *you* more miserable.

Anger may draw others' empathy away from you, even if you happen to be right. I have observed one thing in life: others' opinions and support quietly move away from someone who vehemently and passionately defends his cause. Moreover, if you angrily berate someone and demand immediate admission and correction of a mistake, the other person is likely only to get angry in return. Like a drunkard who entertains others at his own expense, displays of anger hide our words and actions from ourselves but show us to others—only to embarrass us when the spell of anger is over.

Anger does more harm to the person carrying it than to the person targeted. To throw mud, you need to get your hands dirty first. Unfortunately, the harmful chemicals that accompany angry thoughts settle in your body, and cannot be washed out as easily as soil can be washed off your hands.

How can you liberate yourself from anger?

Managing your own anger and managing an angry person in your life, though apparently two different processes, are related. We can manage angry people effectively by learning to manage our own anger while communicating with such people. Communicating with someone who is angry can be challenging, because we cannot always perceive the situation without distortion when we are angry ourselves.

Watch and anticipate your reactions. Understand your responsibility—you have to deal with your own anger. Realize that you are getting irritated or angry. Often this simple realization eludes us because many of us feel guilty about anger, or afraid of what it might mean.

Develop awareness of your anger pattern. Try the following sentence-completion exercise:

- I feel angry when . . .
- When I am angry I tell myself . . .
- Sometimes when I am angry I . . .
- One way I hide my anger is to . . .
- If I could admit that I was angry . . .
- A better way to handle my anger could be . . .

When you watch your thoughts and responses, you learn how your mental software is constituted and how you might need to change. You transform your negative, immobilizing and disempowering thoughts into positive and empowering thoughts.

Keep your cool. Stay relaxed. Identify yourself with a movie screen that, in spite of receiving images of bloodshed, violence and fire from the projector, remains as undisturbed as ever. Instead of picturing yourself as a gasoline tank that explodes when it receives a spark, picture yourself as the cool waters of a lake that quenches the fire of anger. Pay attention to your breathing until it returns to normal.

Ask yourself whether this matter is worth so much anger. Often, mere reflection on this question is enough to lessen your ire. (It is when the roots of anger lie much deeper than the apparent reason that you need to dig up these roots to make the anger subside.)

Before you react to an angry person, try to understand the reasons for his or her behaviour. Place yourself in his or her position. Do not expect him or her to be right and reasonable always; give him or her, as you would like to be given, the freedom to sound unreasonable and wrong from time to time. Understand that every person is the result of what he or she has been born with and gone through. Some things learnt at an early age cannot be unlearnt, even with a lifetime of effort. The wisdom lies in being able to bear what cannot be changed.

Place more importance on what you feel about yourself than on what others feel about you. Try to learn from any criticism you receive. Let people judge you if they have nothing better to do with their time. Do not take away their favourite pastime and the petty satisfaction they derive from it; be generous and let them criticize away. Say to them mentally, 'I don't care what you think of me.' Once your anger has subsided, assume the allegation against you to be true, and see what can you do to improve in that regard.

Do not interrupt the other person when he is talking, even if he is angry. Instead of reacting in kind, let him say all that he wants to say, regardless of whether or not you agree. Allow his anger to flow out and dissipate. Show sympathy (not pity) by being receptive and listening patiently. Most outbursts have their roots in unfulfilled needs and prior incidents; the present incident is usually only a catalyst. Using nods and body language, show that you are listening. This will make the angry person feel understood, and this will help keep him calm, reachable and perhaps sympathetic to your cause.

If you do not agree, there is no need to say so at this stage. Do not try to prove the person wrong. Quietly show him what logic says, or give him any information he does not have, but remember that a person charged with emotion cannot see logic or process new information easily. Accept his right to be angry, and accept him as he is without judging him. Give him the freedom to be wrong. If you have to, learn to mentally disagree with this person's views or approach without ever losing your affection.

Sometimes, apologizing even when you are not at fault can help. This not only dissipates the other person's anger and makes both of you feel lighter and happier, but it patches up the discord—which is far more important than preserving your false ego. You will never lose self-respect by saying, 'I'm sorry,' even when the fault is not yours; it only improves your image in others' eyes. After apologizing, ask the person what *he* wants you to do, rather than pronounce what *you* propose to do. Take corrective action immediately if you are part of his problem, and if you cannot do this, explain why.

When someone is shouting, speak even more softly than you normally do. It will make the other person feel like a fool; he will soon realize that he is the only one shouting.

If you want to express your hurt feelings, refer to them without blaming anyone else directly. Refrain from using the word 'you'—rather, use the word 'I' instead. For example, instead of saying, 'You are unjust, selfish, partial and over-sensitive', which will only inflame the other person, say something to the effect of, 'This bothers me. I feel that my concerns and expectations are not being attended to.'

Walk to the water cooler or filing cabinet across the room. Physical activity helps calm the rush of chemicals in the brain and bring you back to normal. Try this finger technique, too— hold your right middle finger with your left hand if you are being provoked by a male, and your left middle finger with your right hand if your anger is being provoked by a female.

Learn to forgive others. Remind yourself that life is too short for anger. The very fact that you feel hurt means that you care for the person who has made you angry. The realization that you care for this person should make it easier for you to forgive him; it should make you feel lighter, mentally, emotionally and physically. In the end, try to leave him satisfied and in good humour by identifying something good about him and complimenting him for it. This is one way of forgetting the incident and forgiving the person from your heart.

Try sending love and affection instead of anger. Simply ignore how the most difficult people are behaving, and imagine yourself sending out love and affection to them. Pay no attention to the other person's response in this scenario. Gradually make this visualization second nature. If you send out love every time you feel like sending out hatred, you will soon train your brain to run on an altogether different circuitry—one that shall lead you to love, bliss, harmony and fulfilment. You will eventually find it difficult to send hatred at all, or feel a need to take revenge.

Do not try to teach others a lesson. That is not your job. Leave the job of teaching people a lesson to God, as only He can do it justice. Think of the people who sometimes make you angry, and those you think have cheated you in some way. Now realize that they have been playing their parts in the drama enacted to teach *you* the lessons needed for your own spiritual evolution, which includes the art of forgiveness.

Remind yourself of the divine oneness you share with other people. Whenever you meet someone, imagine him or her to be connected to you in some subtle way, and send your love to him or her. This habit will expand your sense of oneness—and people established in oneness cannot be angry with others, because that amounts to being angry with themselves. We all share the same life energy, just as all the electrical equipment on a circuit shares the same electric energy and all the trees in the world have their roots in Mother Earth.

Take responsibility for everything in your life. Whenever you are angry with your circumstances, accept that it was you, knowingly or unknowingly, who created them. Ask yourself, 'What positive lesson can I learn from this? What law of nature is operating?'

Keep a fixed interval every day to jot down all that you are angry about. Be careful when choosing your words; there is a difference between saying, 'I feel cheated' and saying, 'This situation is hopeless.'

Shovel out all your worries and anger. Move your hands as though you were shovelling out a jammed sewer. As you take out the filth, say to yourself, 'I am dipping my shovel into the heap of anger that I carry for [this person or situation]. And here it goes . . . Now, having emptied it, I am now dipping my shovel into the heap of anger that I carry for [that person or situation] . . . And here it goes . . . ' Living well in spite of what you are made to go through is the best lesson you can teach to someone who has wronged you.

Let the accumulated anger within dissipate. Breath into your abdomen for few minutes and be still. When you are available to your feelings and experience them fully, your mind will clear. Imagine that you are dying within an hour. Your mother and/ or father are at your bedside, and you are looking at them intently. This is your last chance to say all that has been unsaid between you—it is now or never. This exercise allows buried and disowned painful feelings to surface and integrate so that the past begins to lose its hold on your present.

Focus on positives instead of being angry with negatives. Do not be *against* war, violence, prostitution, injustice, corruption or anything else. Be *for* peace, dignity for women, justice, integrity and all positive values.

THE FOURTH PRINCIPLE OF REIKI

> *Just for today, I shall do my work sincerely and earn my livelihood honestly.*

You must find your perfect work to find fulfillment in life. Most of us do not realize what work means for our well-being. Work that we love helps us grow mentally, emotionally and spiritually and boosts our self-esteem. People with a high sense of personal worth are more likely to engage themselves in work that gives them an opportunity to express their unique talents, and are more likely to produce high-quality work as well. People with a low sense of self-worth may attract work that weighs them down.

Like seeds, we all have the potential to grow and be successful, but we need the right kind of soil and nourishment. A seed lying on a concrete floor will not grow, despite its inherent potential. Your own unique talents, skills, temperament, commitments, strengths, limitations, interests, intentions and resources suggest certain fields you can excel in (perhaps including, of course, maintaining a home and raising children). Once the right field is found, you hardly feel the 'work' involved; it is effortlessly and spontaneously satisfying.

The degree you earned twenty years ago has very little bearing on what you can do today to satisfy your longings to serve humanity. You have to build on what you did twenty years ago, rather than feel locked into it; and building on it may even mean breaking away from it. Even if you break away, however, subtle learning points gathered from that time still stay with you, and help you work effectively in whatever field you choose.

Each of us is born for a definite purpose. Until you find yours and give your life to it, you fail to begin your adult life. Be sincere in seeking this purpose, because sincerity towards work not meant for you is artificial, laboured, skin-deep and unbeautiful. Stop lamenting whatever economic conditions prevail in the market; look within and listen to your heart. What is your soul crying to do? A recession or dwindling opportunities only reflect the thoughts of scarcity that so many among us are thinking today. When you listen to and trust the cry of your heart, your soul responds by presenting new vistas of opportunity, growth and prosperity in the external world.

How can you find your perfect work?

Lie down on your back and make yourself comfortable. Now ask yourself the following questions:

- *What it is that you are good at?*
- *What is one thing you can do better than most others?*
- *What is one thing you never get tired of doing?*

- *What kind of work would make you feel that you are making the most of your life, that you had accomplished something?*
- *What work would you do if there was no possibility of failure, if you were sure of success?*
- *What would you like to accomplish if you had only one more year to live?*
- *What would you do to pass your time if you had no need to earn money?*

Identify your unique talents and your unique way of expressing them. Identify, too, the human needs they can help you fulfil. Talents are gifts we are born with; skills are abilities we develop through study and practise.

Consider what you love to do. What work have you always dreamed of being involved in? Could you combine two or more of these 'dream jobs' into one? There may be cases in which you love something but do not quite have the skills for it; for instance, a love for the game of cricket does not mean you can become a cricket player. However, you can involve yourself with cricket in a number of other ways: write about it, collect statistics, be a commentator, manufacture cricket bats, organize matches and so on. The idea is to connect your love to the needs of society.

One reason why you might love a particular kind of work is that it offers diversion from your main job—and making this second kind of a work a livelihood might actually squeeze the joy from it. Give it a try on a one-time basis before committing to it, and make sure you have some 'back-up' diversions. Note, too, that doing what we love can make us feel easily hurt in times of failure; be patient and detached. Don't take things too personally.

Consider what you feel strongly about. What would you like to change in the world? What injustices bother you so much that you would like to do something about them? What problems have you been able to overcome? What contribution do you want to make to the world before leaving it? What good things would you like to make sure the world preserves? Have you been ignoring an inner call? When considering your perfect work, do not ask, 'What's in it for me?' Rather, ask, 'How can I serve others, and make a difference in their lives?' Whenever you catch yourself thinking the first question, replace it with the second one.

You may think that 'causes' you feel strongly about will not prove monetarily rewarding, but the satisfaction you derive from working towards them will more than compensate. For example, someone who did not get even a basic formal education as a child for want of money and time may dedicate his life to arranging free education for working children. Discovering yet not fulfilling an inner call can leave a person feeling deprived and disappointed. Mother Theresa, Mahatma Gandhi, Martin Luther King and Nelson Mandela were driven to their missions because these were what gave them satisfaction. Of course, success may come late, and you must be prepared for this.

Your formal education, your area of speciality, your contacts, the organizations you work for, the places you visit and the experiences you develop all have a definite purpose. For example, Mahatma Gandhi endured tremendous hardships in South Africa because the Unmanifest was strengthening him for the challenge of bringing freedom to his motherland. The person who threw him off the train because of his skin colour came into his life so that he would start feeling strongly about fighting discrimination.

When you find your new perfect work, examine your choice. Before you take the plunge and change careers, visualize for a moment that you have already achieved success in your new field. Imagine your daily routine. What are the repercussions for your relationships and your general sense of peace? Are you happy with these changes? Do you feel entirely comfortable with the prospects? Concentrate on your heart chakra, and then on your solar plexus; discomfort in these areas may mean that you need to reconsider the options carefully.

Outgrow your fears of change and struggle. Once you discover your perfect work, you may still lack the courage to leave a safe, secure and familiar job or lifestyle. You may be convinced that you should change your career but doubt your ability to be successful in the new one; or you may like the idea of serving others but fear that it will leave you penniless. Friends and well-wishers may warn you about adverse market conditions and remind you of the neighbour's son who committed suicide for want of a job. The required shift in attitude takes courage, because we are all conditioned to equate unfamiliarity with insecurity. If we look back at our lives, however, we see that everything that was uncertain at one point in time unfolded into security later on. Even before a baby is born, we start worrying about whether it will be healthy enough to survive. When the baby is born and gets sick, we worry that she will not recover. When the child is four, we worry about her admission to a good school, and when she gets admission we start worrying about her grades and her chances of admission to a good college. We then keep our fingers crossed that she will get a good job, and then our worry shifts towards the next phase of life—marriage— and so on . . . this is a never-ending process. At every stage, things clearly work out in everyone's best interests, but we hardly seem to notice this; worry becomes a habit. Struggle is inevitable in life; you can minimize it only with wisdom that you gather from your struggles.

Goethe inspires me with this quote: 'What has not burst forth from your own soul shall never refresh you.'

How should you do your work?

Work with joy and total attention. Once the worker loses awareness of the personal self and becomes *one* with the work, work is *joy*. The greatest moments in our lives are those that make us forget all sense of separateness as an individual—those of being engrossed completely while playing a game like kids, admiring the beauty of a sunset or being in similar state of mind in any other situation. Work can also create such moments for us, if we make our vocation our vacation. The word 'work' has come to be perceived as the antithesis of enjoyment, something we do merely to earn a livelihood. People get tired after a day's work only because they think of 'life' as something to be lived and enjoyed after the workday, rather than during it. When you choose work that you do not tire of doing, you will never have to 'work' a single day; you will be paid for enjoying yourself. And chances are that you shall eventually earn more than you did before.

Work with love and compassion. Let even your smallest and most mundane tasks be expressions of love, signs of sincere gratitude surging from deep within you. When you stir some love into everything you do, you prepare yourself for higher realms of prosperity.

THE FIFTH PRINCIPLE OF REIKI

Just for today, I shall love and respect every living being.

The universe is a seamless oneness of consciousness. Separateness is nothing but a mass hypnotism in which most of us live. A mother can tell that her child needs to be fed, even if the child is not present, by feeling the milk in her breasts. Two decades later, she may feel uneasy and find her thoughts racing to her son abroad, who, it turns out, is in some trouble. How does she know? Because, I suspect, of the interconnectedness of all living beings, which the influence of Newtonian physics has conditioned us to close our eyes to.

Why should we love and respect every living being?

The oneness of the universe is nothing but love. What most of us need to learn is that loving ourselves and loving others are one and the same. Love itself stems from the simple understanding that we are all the same energy, in many different bodies. Reiki is pure love-energy, and that is why we are able to heal another person even if he or she is far away.

Your relationships with everyone and everything else reflect your relationship with yourself. In turn, your relationship with yourself reflects the relationships you had with adults as a child.

The vocabulary with which you scold yourself is probably the same vocabulary they used to scold you all those years ago.

'Usually we attract people who represent our shadow, that aspect of ourselves which we would like to be (or repress) but which we have not yet integrated,' write Bodo Baginski and Shalila Sharamon, authors of *Reiki: The Universal Energy*. Whatever shocks and disturbs us in others has a divine lesson for us: it beckons us to look within and discover what might be similar problems in our own behaviour. When we identify and transform what needs to be transformed in our own character, the other person also begins to change, or moves away from our life. You must change your inner reality to change the external world.

Forgiveness frees us from the prison of pettiness and suffering. It is not weak to forgive; forgiving is a brave act. In fact, it can make the other person feel weak in your presence. You are more likely to make the other person see how foolish his action has been by applying the calm waters of your forgiving silence than by splashing the disturbed waters of angry reaction. Failing to forgive others condemns you to carrying on with your hatred and grudges.

Death shows us what life is for. If you want to know what life is for, imagine looking back at it from the point of death. This will show you unequivocally that every moment is an invaluable opportunity to give and receive love. On your deathbed you will not remember the money and titles that you earned during your life, instead, before your teary eyes, one after the other, will come the blurred faces of the people you loved, those you are leaving behind. You will remember the mistakes you made: you did not love people enough. You did not spend enough time with the people whom you loved. You did not make the contributions to mankind for which your soul yearned; you preferred to play it safe. You wasted many opportunities to serve others, and you did not forgive others or ask for others' forgiveness. Unfortunately, these realizations may come when there is almost no time left to correct your mistakes.

Why do we not love and respect every living being?

We react before we think. We are driven not from within, according to our values, but by our reactions to others' behaviour. 'I will teach him the lesson of his life' appears to have become the common man's motto. Some of us consider our ability to hurt others an index of our supremacy and greatness. The sane alternative of forgiveness takes a back seat; it is considered a sign of timidity and lack of self-respect. If everyone reacts without respecting their own highest values, the world has no desirable values left to emulate.

We seek without what needs to be sought within. We often seek solutions to our problems in the external world, not wanting to confront the fact that all of our miseries originate within. People who hold grudges against others are people who do not want to take the responsibility for their lives; they always hold others responsible for their own unhappiness.

We expect others to behave, and things to happen, just as we want them to. You must surrender this expectation and desire— let people behave the way they have learnt to behave, and let things happen the way the universe wants them to happen. We must be grateful to the universe for all that is good *and* bad in our lives, for it is all programmed for our best interests.

We fail to distinguish between love and attachment. In love there is no ownership; in attachment there is nothing but ownership. Love considers and respects the changing nature of the universe, while attachment sticks to the illusion of permanence. Love accepts and lets others flow with their lives, while attachment does not tolerate change. Love has no unreasonable expectations, while attachment seeks to ensure that everything runs according to expectation. With love you grow; with attachment you wither and waste. The latter breeds lust, while the former frees one from it.

We are attached to money, material possessions, places, property, buildings, security, people, perfection, our past, our bodies, our opinions (and others' opinions of them), our image (mainly in others' eyes), our beliefs and ideas and our desires to win and be right all the time. With so many attachments, it is almost impossible to feel the love within, for love accepts no bondage—it needs space and freedom. Examine these attachments, and observe and catch yourself whenever you find yourself thinking, speaking and acting because of any one of them. Do not condemn or justify them or yourself; just notice it and let it go.

How to liberate the fountain of love within?

Stop identifying yourself with merely your physical body. We tend to think that we are our bodies. With this belief begins the illusion of separation, and the belief that everything is scarce. Other people's achievements appear to be at our cost, since we see the world's resources as finite and limited. We stop believing anything intangible, and we start feeling that we are islands—disconnected from every other being and every other thing.

Because our real being is omnipresent, omnipotent and omniscient, we want to be present everywhere—in everyone's mind—hence our desire to be famous, powerful and knowledgeable. Because our real nature is *ananda,* or bliss, we are always seeking pleasure. What a paradox! In our search for pleasure, we become greedy, yet we are only seeking what we already are.

Do not gossip. Just for a few days do not say anything about anyone who is not present. Do not talk about people who annoy you, or even those who please you; do not complain about how others are behaving. Spend your words as you would spend money. Do not speak unnecessarily; preserve energy. You will be surprised by how little we actually need to speak, and how foolishly we keep wasting our energy. It is absolutely essential to establish inner silence, as God waits for you to calm down before he speaks to you.

In the same vein, *shift your focus from what is missing in the other person to whatever you find admirable.* This shift will dramatically improve your relationships. Realize that every moment and every being are expressions of divine love. Learn to see beyond the 'dirt on the surface' so you can concentrate on this collective divine. Others cannot harm you if the script that you have co-authored with the Latent Oneness does not allow it; you are bound to get what you deserve, which is whatever is in your best interests. You will immediately see the difference in your peace and energy levels.

Remember that you get out of life whatever you put into it. What you do to others is what you do to yourself; identify yourself with others and seek for them what you seek for yourself. Keep others' wishes in mind while pursuing fulfilment of your own. When birds, insects and ants cause problems in your day-to-day life, find a way to get rid of them that respects their wish to live, since this is what you wish for yourself as well. Similarly, do not seek solace in the punishment of people who seem to have wronged you; just try to move away from them without thwarting their own wishes. Never be tempted to seek harm for others; this will not lessen your suffering.

Transform your lust into love. When you transform lust into intense and unconditional love, you will find that others shower love upon you instead of using you for their ends. How do you perceive others? What thoughts sprout within your mind when you see or meet a person of the opposite sex? Do you see others as physical objects that can be used to fulfil your needs, physical or otherwise? Do you visualize using them in a crude way? If you are not sure, start watching yourself. Such thoughts degrade ourselves, others and God as mere objects. We are not objects; we are divine beings meant to appreciate our divinity by sharing our collective ocean of pure, unconditional love.

Every time you catch yourself having lustful thoughts ('How can I use him/her?'), replace them with thoughts of pure love ('How can I express my love for him/her, devoid of all expectation and regardless of all opinion?'). Imagine yourself blessing the person mentally: picture a white beam of love-light shooting out from your heart chakra and enveloping him or her completely. Say a prayer for him or her.

Do not be tempted to teach others a lesson—except by your own example. Someone who has never seen good human behaviour cannot be expected to exhibit it.

Redefine your goals in terms of giving. Giving is a great value. In the early years of my career, I used to get very touchy about whether or not I got my due, whether or not others treated me with respect. One day I realized that this attitude kept the reins of my well-being in others' hands. I decided to reframe my concerns in terms of giving. Instead of asking, 'What can I get, and how can I get it?' I now ask, 'What can I give, and how can I give it?' My life has miraculously changed for the better since that day. Friends often tell me I am undermining my self-respect and surrendering my rights too meekly, but self-respect does not depend on what you get; it depends on what you *give* to others and to society. Look around and you will see that the happiest and the most inspiring people are not those who hanker after material goods and rewards but those who focus their lives on *giving*. Mother Theresa was a great human being because she did not have time to think about herself . . . by focusing entirely on giving, she got all that she would not have got had she focused on getting. The surest way of getting is to *give* to others what you want for yourself.

Use visualization. Lie down on your back. Relax your body through yoga nidra or any other progressive relaxation technique. Think of someone you love very much, and let the feelings of love gather and overflow. Now imagine these feelings as a shining, laser-like beam of love-energy shooting out of your heart. Imagine it splitting in two, then four, then eight as it moves out and forms a network of love-beams engulfing your home, locality, state, country, continent, the world, the galaxies and the universe. Imagine that as the beam network splits into more and more beams, it multiplies in love-energy intensity as well; and that as this happens, you feel a similar corresponding upsurge in your own feelings of love. Imagine that every living being is getting soaked in your love-energy, overflowing with love, happiness, joy and prosperity and feeling ecstatic about it. Imagine each one of them thanking the Latent Oneness for your shower of love.

Stay at this a little while before you begin imagining the return journey of the love-energy beam. Once you start, see the beams getting more and more powerful as they merge into half their numbers, one-fourth their numbers and so forth, until finally the last but most powerful beam comes back into your heart and overwhelms you with its energy. Imagine the love-energy being transformed into all that you want for yourself, and feel the ecstasy of limitless abundance. Keep this exercise a secret.

We now come to the end of our discussion on the spirit of Reiki. 'Great principles!' you think. 'But how can I really remember so much and use them in my life?'

Knowing is not enough. These principles need to be practised day in and day out; you need to live them every moment of your life. Often knowledge serves no other purpose but to make us feel guilty for not being able to practise it. The intensity of your desire to live by these principles shall make the rest easy.

I suggest that you divide your day into five equal parts and focus on learning just one principle during each part. Begin the day by giving Reiki to a visualization that you are practising each principle with perfect success. Before going to sleep, review your progress in each of the five areas and draw lessons, if any, for better implementation the next day. After forty days, switch the principle to be followed in each slot, and keep doing so until you have practised each principle in each slot. Keep a diary to record your progress, your stumbling blocks, your weaknesses, your failures and what you have learnt from them. Make plans for overcoming them, and stay on the path. If you miss a day, make it a point not to miss on two consecutive days.

The first few days will indicate the difficulties and challenges involved; it is often difficult to overcome and unlearn deep-rooted bad habits. To make it easier, use the Swish technique (see 'Affirmation and Attitude' in Chapter 4) in conjunction with the Reiki symbols. When you replace your initial visualization of behaving undesirably with that of behaving according to the five principles of Reiki, start mentally drawing symbols on the latter. As you persevere, the principles will gradually become second nature.

Epilogue

Staying on the Path

Having finished this book, you have proved your interest in improving the quality of your life. Congratulations! However, you still need to prove something more important than mere interest—your *commitment* to making Reiki your way of life. So what you are going to do now? Some of you may just evaluate this as a good book (or otherwise) and rush to purchase another one to pass your time. Though amusing you has not been the purpose of this book, the truth is that most people opt for just this—they do not use the knowledge they are empowered with. Instead of using their knowledge and awareness to grow in all areas of their lives, they prefer to pass through life somehow with minimal proactive effort, often using various kinds of amusements (including books) to escape the uncomfortable truths of their lives. Still, I would estimate that more than ninety-five per cent of those who become Reiki channels or learn any similar self-growth technique eventually stop using it, at least on a regular basis. *Results come from doing, not merely from knowing.*

Great self-growth techniques like Reiki, along with great gurus and great books, are like restaurant menus: they hold promise for your nourishment, as long as you are hungry enough to use them. Today we are living in a 'turn-key' culture. We outsource all our responsibilities to experts for a fee. We hire a coach to teach our child lawn tennis; we hire event managers to organize our weddings; and we outsource our spiritual growth to some spiritual organization or guru or 'ism', not realizing that while others can serve us the food, they cannot chew, swallow or assimilate it for us.

One common feature in all successful people who strive towards their full potential or divinity is a superior determination—a burning desire to stay on the path and never lose sight of the ultimate goal.

To keep your fire of intention burning:

Love yourself enough. Life is very, very precious—it is a rare opportunity to realize our divinity. Yet this opportunity slips out of our hands every single minute, the same way water does. Still, many of us live life as if there is another one saved in the bank. Stand in front of the mirror every morning and smile. Say to yourself that this day is never going to return, and you are going to live it to the hilt so you never need to regret it. Tell yourself that you love yourself completely, and feel it very deeply. Tell yourself that you value yourself immensely, and hence will not lose this priceless opportunity for spiritual growth through the infallible technique of Reiki.

Remember that you can take away only what your spirit can consume and carry with it—spiritual growth! You can't take anything that you buy, eat or wear into the next world; these will not make any value addition to the 'real you' that survives your physical death. Investment of both time and money in your spiritual growth is the wisest investment you can make, for its fruits are permanent in a way that your body is not.

Doubt your doubts. The universe has no purpose but to fulfil your wishes and bring you what you want—but the universe gives first to those who trust in its intention to grant people their wishes. With unconditional self-love, unquestionable belief in your dreams, unwavering determination and an infallible technique like Reiki, nothing can stop you from fulfilling your dreams. Reiki may not fulfill your wants (which stem from your ego), but it will certainly help you fulfil your needs (which stem from the spiritual purpose you were born for).

Don't let the whispers of the important things in life be lost in the cacophony of 'urgent' things. We always find time for what we find important, but what we deem important can change once we know our real needs. Many of us cannot distinguish between what is important and what is urgent.

Often people blame their irregularity and derailments from Reiki on external circumstances. One friend confided in me, 'Although I have learnt Reiki, I am not able to do it regularly because of endless interruptions. Often, just when I settle down to do it, there is a phone call, or the doorbell rings and I need to entertain unexpected guests, or the dhobi comes to the door asking for his payment, or the sweeper asks for the garbage bin.' She says she has thought of taking the phone off the hook but fears she might miss an urgent call. On being reminded that she *had* done Reiki for twenty-one days before in spite of all these things, she admitted that at that time there was a compulsion (pain in her knees), but that when there is no compulsion, she is driven mostly by the dictates of the external world rather than inner resolve or self-discipline.

Whereas urgent things catch our immediate attention and demand that we act upon them, important things do not; we need to choose to act upon them. If we do not go for a morning walk or meditate or do yoga, Reiki or any other such thing that will aid in our all-around growth, we will never in our lives be questioned or forced to do these things. But if we consider them important, we will find a way to include them in our daily schedule.

Earmark an appropriate time slot and venue for Reiki. Then just bring yourself to the right place at the right time, every single day. Do not be at any other place at the appointed time. You may need to go to bed early in order to steal a big enough time slot for Reiki in the morning, for mornings alone are all yours. Evenings are usually uncertain; unexpected guests may turn up, and so forth. If you do not put first things first in your life, you will fail to find any time for them throughout out the day, in spite of your best intentions.

Often people do not think deeply about the effort and time required on a daily basis for something like Reiki. When the initial attraction or novelty of this new healing system wears off, they can no longer bring themselves to practise day in and day out, and they eventually just give up. Before adopting a regimen like Reiki, make sure you will be able to make time for it, and make sure you accept the whole routine—do not take up Reiki just because a family member or friend is doing it.

When you are about to miss Reiki on a particular day, reschedule it immediately for another time that day. Maybe you can do it while waiting in a queue or commuting to a meeting or during the time you would have spent reading the newspaper or watching TV. If you must miss an entire day for external reasons, vow that you absolutely will not miss Reiki the next day. Make it a rule never to miss your Reiki session on two consecutive days.

Do not let small chunks of time go waste, either. Use these for affirmations, visualizations, contemplation, prayers or Reiki. If you take ten minutes to fall asleep, consider going to bed twenty minutes before the usual time, and lo! You have added to your day another half hour of Reiki. Get in the habit of identifying and stealing small chunks of time at appropriate times of the day.

Keep a journal to record the regularity with which you practise Reiki. Every day, note how much time you spent giving Reiki to yourself or to others, in which positions, what you observed and what you learned. Did you receive intuitive guidance? Think about which areas of your life you need to be happier about, and ask yourself how you can use Reiki to accomplish that.

Recording your progress on the path brings awareness of how you are spending your time. You might be surprised to find that you are not as regular in following your practise as you think, and that, like most people, you waste major chunks of your day on fruitless activities. You will then realize the hollowness of the excuse that you do not have enough time for Reiki. The sheer amount of time you waste is likely to wake you up. Ask yourself throughout the day: 'Is this activity worth my time? Does it gel with my life purpose? Will it advance me on my path? Does it show my respect and love for the God that resides within me and is, in fact, the real me? A few moments or years from now, will I regret or cherish having spent time on this activity?'

Do not envision a dichotomy between 'spiritual hours' and 'non-spiritual' or 'casual' hours. Some people find it satisfying to do their sadhana during a specific time of day, leaving them free to do whatever they consider mundane, material, sensual or unspiritual for the rest of the day. Never forget that our spiritual growth is not indicated by how many hours we devote to our sadhana, but by the level of divine awareness (or spiritual quality) these hours infuse into the rest of the day.

Seek to improve yourself on all fronts, for problems are opportunities for spiritual growth. Creative thinking simply means realizing that there is no particular virtue in doing things the way they have always been done. If you want different results, you cannot continue to live your life the way you have been living it. Unlike hunger for food, hunger to learn new things (and improve the old) increases as you satisfy it. You may feel that you have no desire to improve, but if you spot even a single area or problem in your life that interests you, try to satisfy its hunger with Reiki. Once the hunger for growth crosses the boundaries from one area to another, there will be no end to it. Education is essentially the ability to direct the will towards the right goals.

Whether you are (or want to be) a salesman or a scientist, an engineer or a doctor, an artist or a critic, a politician or a social worker, a teacher or a philosopher, a journalist or an administrator, you can always use Reiki, its principles and its techniques creatively to scale new heights.

Stay connected to God. Give thanks to God when you manage to stick to the path, as even the smallest accomplishments of ours come from God's grace. If you get derailed, pray for guidance and for help getting back on track. Sometimes nothing seems to work; day-to-day issues keep cropping up and life seems to get sucked into unavoidable, time-consuming trivialities, addictions, emergencies and formalities. There never seems to be light at the end of the tunnel. Do not give up—you cannot make your problems smaller, but you can always make yourself bigger than they are.

Commit to transforming your life with this book. Re-read the book to select material you would particularly like to work on. I want you to be obsessed with the idea of using Reiki and its principles to improve the way you live your life. Only this obsession to improve will ensure that what you have learnt in this book does not get lost as temporary intellectual entertainment.

There is a Chinese saying:

I hear, I forget.
I see, I remember.
I do, I understand.

So far you have only heard (read), so you might *forget*.

Your next step is to see: to constantly apply what you have learnt to real life, observing situations where you can use Reiki to obtain desired results. The use of Reiki is limited only by your own imagination. Visualize the use of Reiki techniques in the appropriate areas; this way you will *remember* how Reiki can help you.

Then *do* it. Put into practice today one of the techniques you picked up and visualized yesterday, and you will *understand*. Keep at it, day after day.

Just one caution: while heading down your new path, you may sometimes appear to be moving in the wrong direction. Remember it is often necessary to go south for a while in order to journey north. What appears to be nothing but chaos may, in fact, be an essential rough patch on your journey towards order.

With these powerful strategies, you can now enjoy your romance with Reiki, and get wedded to it for eternity!

My unconditional love and best wishes are with you.

Appendix

Becoming a Master Teacher

Hawayo Takata proclaimed that only those who are willing to give up everything in their lives should take a Reiki mastership attunement. What she meant was that if you want to be a Reiki teacher, you must let go of your old ways. You cannot climb a staircase if you are unwilling to let go of the railing; you cannot fill a glass that is already full. Reiki facilitates personal growth only in proportion to one's willingness to let go of old ways. Perfection is by no means the pre-requisite for becoming a master, but you must be willing to accept your shortcomings and to grow at all costs. Everyone is moving towards the same goal in life, and although the paths may be different, each path is perfect for the person who follows it. Someone who understands this and refrains from judging others can start down the spiritual path to becoming a Reiki master.

As a would-be master, you must learn and thoroughly practise the methods of all levels of attunement. Try to attend the Reiki seminars of other masters and remember the best aspects of each. Eventually you will learn how to relate to students effectively, and pick up other subtle essentials as well. You must be a keen observer in order to clarify the minutest doubts raised in your own mind or by others. You may want to jot down questions about first- and second-degree Reiki as they arise, and then discuss them with your own master or research them in literature. The longer and more sincere your association with your master, and the keener your observation, the more you will benefit from this training.

A teacher is one who shares knowledge on the basis of his or her experience, so you can be a good teacher only if you spend a great deal of time over a prolonged period getting first-hand experience of Reiki's short-term and long-term effects. You must spend time in silence to grow sensitive enough to receive intuitive wisdom, and you must constantly observe the thoughts and sensations that arise while practising Reiki. Often guidance comes in the form of intuitive thoughts during Reiki sessions, and following this guidance may lead you to new findings that you can share with others—remembering, of course, that they may represent merely your own perception of Reiki, not the universal truth. Prolonged practice of Reiki makes one sensitive to its laws. The right attitude is that of striving but never feeling that you have arrived.

Most people who become Reiki master teachers have also followed some spiritual discipline. You must know the limitations of Reiki so that you do not, in your enthusiasm, propagate unrealistic claims. (Inflating people's expectations might cause them to lose faith in Reiki's efficacy.) Let people make up their minds about Reiki's efficacy on the basis of their own experiences. Their faith might be slow to grow, but it will be concrete and realistic. You should continue acquiring knowledge of anatomy, psychology, physiology, psychotherapy, counseling, holistic healing, chakras, aural sheaths and so forth, but refrain from giving medical advice—even if you feel sure of it—unless you are also a formally trained and qualified medical practitioner.

The laws of nature do not change with time. You cannot give your student or client more than he is prepared to take, or force him to take it at any particular time. You can only inspire students to ask more of life. Those who do not expect much from life will not feel inspired to give it their best; and when they do not give it their best, their dreams remain only dreams. If your client does not expect to be healed, he will obstruct his healing process. If he is not ready to do his part of the work— to learn to learn lessons from his ailments, to change his thought patterns, attitudes or diet—he may simply invite his ailments back. Neither Reiki nor the Reiki master can do his work, just as no one can eat on someone else's behalf in order to nourish him. As a master teacher you must be very clear on this, and must not encourage spoon-feeding. You must take full responsibility for everything in your own life, and teach others by your own example.

Many truth-seekers are not aware that in the name of truth they actually seek almost everything but the truth—ranging from approval and recognition to money, security and publicity. A truth-seeker does not need to shun the world for the sake of truth; he must simply detach himself somewhat, and thus be better prepared to change his ways and beliefs for the sake of truth. As a real teacher, you must seek lessons in everything, and you will find them—because God provides what you seek in proportion to your hunger. Reiki does not make you divine; it just makes you sensitive to your inherent divinity. It also makes you aware of your own hypocrisy, shortcomings and other imperfections, and helps you accept them gracefully—not as a source of brooding and nursing guilt, but as a means of understanding and transcending them.

One sign of progress on the path is that you start accepting people, events and situations as they are. You are deeply content with yourself, yet you do not feel superior to others in any way. You catch yourself thinking, 'Everything is the way it ought to be.' You start seeing yourself and everything else not in isolation but as a part of an all-encompassing larger reality. You do not get angry if others disagree with your point of view; you let people say or believe as they please without offending you. You become a Reiki master when—alongside your own ceaseless, indefatigable march down the path of spirituality—you show infinite patience with everything and everyone.

To be a good teacher, you must look back at your life and ask what pieces of information, inspiration and practise have helped you become what you are today. You can then ensure that you provide your students with all of that, in addition to everything else they will need to become even better masters themselves.

ETHICS AND GUIDELINES

Do not reduce demands on students in order to get more from them. An effective master does not hesitate to emphasize that complacency begets obsolescence. The greatest obstacle on the path of Reiki (as on any other path) is irregularity in practising. Nothing else, not even intelligence, can compensate for regularity. Students must be warned: 'You must make time for Reiki every day. Are you prepared to do that? Will you do it every day just as you brush your teeth and take a bath? If you cannot, then go away, and come back only when you are prepared to do that. Reiki is serious business meant for serious people who are ready to pay the price in terms of time, money, determination and discipline.'

Begin to *be* what you present yourself as. It is a law of Nature that you will get what you deserve, when you deserve it—not before that. The closer you get to the image you want to showcase, the more legitimacy you will attain as a master and the more chances you will be given to serve Reiki. Be careful while thinking or talking to others—watch for any tendency to 'show off', particularly as a spiritual person, such as hinting about your spiritual powers in cleverly concealed words. If you remember that you are as ordinary as everyone else, you ensure yourself harmonious spiritual development.

Do not hesitate to ask for energy exchange. Reiki is not social work. The principles of Reiki are more important than the goody-goody image you may wish to earn and carry forth. It is easy not to ask for energy exchange, but Dr Mikao Usui discovered that failing to do so is counterproductive for both the giver and the receiver of Reiki. Reiki should not be diluted by being given to those who are not ready to pay the price. There is no need to feel guilty about spending the money you receive, though, of course, it is always a good idea to donate part of it to charitable institutions.

As a master, you must not make the mistake of propagating Reiki as social work. The circumstances people find themselves in are the results of their own choices in thought, speech and action. Until they realize this and take responsibilty for their lives by changing their inner responses to external realities, your help will not be much help. Let others say that you are practising Reiki for the sake of others, but do not nurture illusions in this regard. Know that you are really doing it for yourself—because *you* want happiness, excitement, satisfaction, relief from guilt and so forth.

Once you see that giving free Reiki is not social work but an attempt to satisfy a hidden, unresolved longing on your own part, you take the first step towards identifying that longing. Giving free Reiki without introspection may deprive you of knowing your own motivations, and hence of knowing yourself. In addition, free Reiki is wasted on someone who may have come to take it only because it was free. Free Reiki encourages the dilution of norms and standards handed down by the great masters, because on a subconscious level it absolves the master of any responsibility to maintain high (or even any) standards.

Decline any patient who demands a guarantee. Asking for a guarantee often shows a general sense of distrust towards everything, and may actually be one of the attitudinal reasons for the inquirer's problems. Politely explain why you cannot guarantee results. Paradoxically, Reiki works best when both the healer and the healee are detached from the results. Make it very clear that you can guarantee only your sincerity and commitment. Some people may ask whether you have treated other patients with the same disease; in this case, clarify that it is not you who heals but Reiki, and that even if you have helped cure someone in the past, you cannot guarantee the same results for this person. Healing demands commitment not only on the part of the healer but also on the part of the healee.

Becoming a teacher does not mean bidding farewell to healing sessions. A teacher goes on becoming a better one by providing regular healings, both to himself and to others. What separates teachers from other channels is their combination of striking humility and extensive practical experience with Reiki. A Reiki master is not someone who has 'mastered' Reiki but one who has surrendered his life to its spirit. He does not govern

Reiki, but, rather, lovingly offers himself to be governed by her.

YOUR INITIATION

It is best to ascertain the contents of your Reiki teacher initiation beforehand. Your master should be able to tell you what your certification will qualify you to do; some masters teach you how to attune people only for Reiki I or Reiki II, which means added expenditure on your part to learn to teach Reiki III in a separate session. You should also ask how much opportunity you will have to practise attuning others, as this is what you will have to do independently later on. Look for a teacher who will give you enough time and support to make you a confident teacher in your own right.

Apart from practice sessions with your teacher, you should spend a great deal of time at home practising attunements on teddy bears or on volunteers already attuned to the level of Reiki you are practising. (Additional attunements can only improve them as channels.) Rehearsals for seminars can enhance your confidence level; you may want to jot down an outline of your lecture, tape your lecture, listen to it and make improvements. Pray to Reiki for inspiration to give your best to your students. Pray for success. And above all, visualize success.

Check your attitude—do you really want to help others, or do you just want to attract more students to get more money? The attitude you carry will decide the number and the kind of students you attract. The more you give to others, the more you take for yourself. Do not look at your students as future competitors.

CONDUCTING ATTUNEMENTS

- The attunement room should be clean, and should have as little furniture as possible. It should be absolutely calm and quiet, and relatively dark. Prior to attunements, you should clean the room spiritually with Reiki symbols and burn some incense sticks.

- The room should be properly ventilated (short of drawing the curtains, as this lets in too much light) and should be kept at a comfortable temperature, as it will get warmed up by Reiki and remain so afterwards. You own body may also feel hot and tired after attunements.
- Wash your hands soon after each attunement. Do not conduct attunements if you feel more than slightly ill.
- Wear loose, light clothing. If possible, remove your rings, wristwatch, wallet, belt and other accessories.
- Handle the attunement bells (about which you will learn during attunement) with respect.

These instructions are by no means exhaustive; you will learn others in your initiation.

INSTRUCTIONS TO GIVE THOSE BEING ATTUNED

Before attunements, you should advise patients:

- to wear loose, light clothing and remove rings, wristwatches, wallets and other accessories.
- not to keep their hands too loose or too tight when they are asked to hold them in the namaskar mudra during the attunement process. The tips of all the fingers should be at the same level to facilitate the master in holding the patient's hands.
- not to open their eyes or talk during the entire attunement process.
- to go back to the seminar room and again lie quietly after the attunement is over.
- to understand that aggravation of symptoms does not occur in every case (lest they imagine such aggravation even in its absence).

It is a sheer joy to see yourself transfer the power of Reiki onto others through attunements, and then to guide students in its use. Think of the chain you have triggered off: these students will provide Reiki to themselves, relatives, friends and others, and some of them may become teachers themselves and widen the circle even further.

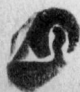